The Couple's Guide to In Vitro Fertilization

D0094363

The Couple's Guide to In Vitro Fertilization

EVERYTHING YOU NEED TO KNOW TO MAXIMIZE
YOUR CHANCES OF SUCCESS

LIZA CHARLESWORTH

Da Capo
LIFE
LONG

A Member of the
Perseus Books Group

Designed by Lisa Kreinbrink
Set in 10 point New Baskerville by The Perseus Books Group

Cataloging-in-Publication data for this book is
available from the Library of Congress.

First Da Capo Lifelong Books edition 2004
ISBN 0-7382-0897-3

Published by Da Capo Lifelong Books
A Member of the Perseus Books Group
http://www.dacapopress.com

Da Capo Lifelong books are available at special discounts for bulk
purchases in the U.S. by corporations, institutions, and other
organizations. For more information, please contact the Special
Markets Department at the Perseus Books Group, 11 Cambridge
Center, Cambridge, MA 02142, or call (800) 255-1514 or (617) 252-
5298, or e-mail special.markets@perseusbooks.com.

2 3 4 5 6 7 8 9—08 07 06 05 04

To my husband, Justin Martin,
by my side every step of the journey

Contents

ॐ

Introduction:
Journey to Babyland
༄

Dear Reader,

Because you're reading this book, it's safe to assume that you're contemplating in vitro fertilization. Perhaps you're perusing these pages after a year of carefully timed lovemaking failed to result in a pregnancy—"just in case" you'll need the treatment down the road. Perhaps your OB/GYN referred you to a fertility practice, mentioning the process as a possible option. Or maybe you've already had a battery of tests and been told by a reproductive endocrinologist that your best, or only, chance of getting pregnant is IVF. Regardless of your personal story, chances are you're frustrated and confused. Quite possibly, too, you're mad at your body for letting you down. After all, everywhere you turn women are either glowingly pregnant or cooing into prams. At least, that's how it seems.

I remember those feelings well. Despite the fact that nearly 10 percent of U.S. couples struggle with some degree of infertility, the inability to conceive can be isolating and downright depressing. After years of meticulous birth control to prevent pregnancies, the rules are suddenly turned on their heads. Now, the point is to *get pregnant* at any cost. When the desire for a baby strikes, it strikes with a vengeance. I still recall the day my husband and I popped the cork on a bottle of champagne and decided to start "trying." At 35, our wild oats were sown. We had a comfy apartment in Manhattan, complete with a sunny spare room just the right size for a nursery. But a year came and went and the room remained empty. And my relaxed, "let-it-happen-when-it-happens" mind-set morphed into a full-fledged campaign to achieve a pregnancy.

It was time to get serious. After a lengthy exam, my OB/GYN pronounced me "just fine." My husband, however, was a different story. Turns out, his sperm count was precariously low. Bingo. We'd discovered our problem. So began our initiation into the wide world of fertility treatments. Following eight frustrating stabs at intrauterine insemination, we decided to pursue IVF. Then, after six months on the waiting list of a prominent New York clinic, we landed, like Magellan, in the wood-paneled office of a top in-vitro doctor. But the journey didn't end there. Our quest for a baby spanned four years and included one failed—and pricey—cycle of in vitro, one miscarriage, and an emergency thyroidectomy that put me out of commission for several months.

During that period, life went on. I worked, hung out with friends, scrubbed the bathtub, read, and baked chocolate-chip cookies. To the untrained eye, it was business as usual. But I felt like I was barely holding it together. Still, a little voice inside my head nudged me to keep going. So I did, completing a second cycle of IVF in March of 2001, then anxiously awaiting the results of my pregnancy test. When the staff nurse called to say that it looked like I was pregnant with not one but *two* babies, I was so elated I practically hit the ceiling. Today, my twin sons—Dash and Theo—are full-fledged toddlers, knee-deep in the terrible twos. Toy cars clutter the living room, jelly handprints adorn the walls, juice cups get hurled from cribs in protest of naptime ... and my husband and I take none of this for granted. Parenthood was our deepest wish.

To be honest, the goal to have children was the toughest challenge I ever set for myself. IVF required me to be patient *and* proactive. It also introduced me to a host of industrial-strength emotions I didn't know I had—namely, anger, jealousy, sadness, frustration, and, thankfully, determination. But my story isn't unique. Many women and men find such treatments to be the most demanding chapter of their lives. That's where this book comes in. As I roamed the twisty path of in vitro fertilization, I asked myself, Why isn't there a great guidebook on the subject? And I vowed to write one.

Here it is—I hope.

My purpose in creating this book is to provide a friendly road map to help you navigate your journey to the baby you so desire and deserve. No question, coping with infertility can be a struggle, but with knowledge and emotional support, it can be overcome. The fact is the majority of people who try IVF have babies after one to three cycles. Readers, like you, should feel very enthusiastic about the odds. I worked hard to communicate my optimism as well as to make the content relevant and understandable—writing in the language of real people, not doctor-ese. In the chapters that follow, you'll find statistics to help assess your specific chances of success, tips for taking fertility tests, and suggestions to determine if IVF is the best choice for you. I've provided practical information on the important topics of managing emotions, making treatments affordable, picking the perfect medical practice, and, if necessary, locating an egg donor or gestational surrogate. In addition, I've included a thorough description of the entire process—from the first shot of Lupron to the culminating pregnancy test.

These pages also include dozens of observations from people intimately involved in IVF. During the course of my research, I spoke to several leading fertility doctors. Without exception, they were generous and helpful. But the folks who taught me the most about in vitro were those who'd actually gone through it. You'll find their pithy comments and sage advice woven throughout the text. Talking with this diverse group of women—and men—was my favorite part of the job. They were wise, articulate, always honest, and often funny. They were creative, resilient, courageous, and inspiring. Although their names have been changed to allow them to speak with candor, their stories will likely hit home. Helen, a 39-year-old homemaker, and her husband, Harvey, turned to IVF after cancer treatments compromised her ovaries. Today, they're the proud parents of preteen twin girls obsessed with soccer and MTV. After several failed cycles, Belinda, a 29-year-old attorney, and her husband,

Todd, traveled 2,000 miles to seek treatments from one of the best reproductive endocrinologists in the business. It worked: Their strawberry-blond son is nearly three!

Then there's Jillian. With the support of her partner, Ted, and a tight-knit family, this publicist became a new mom at the age of 48—thanks to a miracle egg from an anonymous donor. "Dealing with in vitro was huge," she recounts. "There was so much to do, so much uncertainty. Some days I had major meltdowns. But then a ray of hope would poke through the clouds and give me the energy to persevere. Now that the treatments are over, my baby's a daily reminder to stay hopeful."

Yes, there is much reason to be hopeful. To date, hundreds of thousands of people have brought home babies thanks to in vitro fertilization. And the odds get better with each passing year. It's my dream that this book will fulfil the role of a trusted friend, supporting you through the process and helping you realize your dream of parenthood very soon.

Warmly,
Liza Charlesworth

Chapter 1

The Facts on IVF

The Cry
Heard Around the World

A few minutes before midnight on July 25, 1978, a baby girl with clear blue eyes and a hearty cry was born in Oldham, England. Weighing in at 5 pounds, 12 ounces, her arrival represented a watershed event for her parents—and everyone else. That baby, named Louise Brown, was the first ever to have been conceived outside the body, a fact not lost on the world. Newspapers from New York to Nagasaki trumpeted the arrival of the first "test-tube" baby. Doctors, medical ethicists, coworkers, and couples heatedly discussed the topic. Was the baby normal? Would this procedure cause her serious medical problems down the road? Was sex for procreation's sake a thing of the past? Could *they* take advantage of this amazing technology? The world watched and waited as Louise—surprise, surprise—grew into a happy and healthy adult.

This miracle baby brought about by Dr. Patrick Steptoe and Dr. Robert Edwards was an instant sensation. However, she was no overnight success. The determined doctors had toiled for more than 10 years and oversaw 80 failed attempts—on a number of infertile women—before finally achieving a pregnancy. Their exciting news set off a flurry of IVF activity worldwide, including the 1981 birth of the very first American in-vitro baby, Elizabeth Carr. She came courtesy of the Jones Institute in Norfolk, Virginia, the very first IVF practice in the States. But such victories were few and far between. The procedure was really only appropriate for women with tubal obstructions. Plus it was expensive, labor-intensive, and hit or miss to say the least. Think of closing your eyes and throwing a dart at a small bulls-eye on the side of a barn; those were pretty much the odds of achieving an IVF pregnancy in those days. Doctors were working in the dark and had few colleagues with whom to share ideas. In the 1980s, the handful of lucky couples to do IVF and bring home babies either became local celebrities or chose to keep mum so that their children would not be stigmatized. Amy, a 47-year-old homemaker and mom of early IVF twins, chose the latter: "It was not something you talked about back then, because some people looked at your wonderful kids and saw a science project. I wanted them to fit in."

When the '90s rolled around, however, in vitro began to hit its stride. Although the process was still a bit wobbly, steady progress *was* being made. Doctors were getting more skillful at nurturing eggs and successfully fertilizing them. Frozen and thawed embryos were starting to result in pregnancies. And, in 1992, a 62-year-old gave birth to a baby boy using an egg donated from another woman! Fertility was fast becoming a hot field and a genuine calling for the sort of physicians who wanted to make a real difference in their patients' lives. Suddenly, IVF clinics were cropping up across the country. There were hospital and university programs and even a scattering of private practices—each offering a ray of hope to those willing to commit to as many as 10 attempts and, often, tens of thousands of dollars for a slim chance of bringing home a baby.

Flash forward to the present. To date, more than one million babies have been born thanks to IVF. Over time, the technology has evolved in much the same way as the automobile. Through slow and steady tinkering, the state of the art has vastly improved. As a result, it has become more widely sought out and, in response, more available. Now there are options and customization to meet the varied needs of people across the country. Today, the treatment has become almost commonplace—albeit costly—with more than 400 centers nationwide and success rates for the very best in-vitro practices approaching 50 percent per cycle. A couple pursuing 10 cycles is a rarity; if it's going to work, it usually takes three tries or fewer. These days, IVF serves not only women with tubal obstructions, but those with endometriosis, polycystic ovarian syndrome, poor egg quality, irregular menstrual cycles, antibody issues, recurrent miscarriages, and unexplained infertility. It's also a highly effective treatment when a male partner's sperm count is low or seemingly nonexistent. In addition, it offers promise to couples with a predisposition to devastating illnesses, such as sickle-cell anemia or cystic fibrosis. A process called Preimplantation Genetic Diagnosis (PGD) enables doctors to examine the embryos and transfer only those that do not contain these harmful genes.

Fertility Fact: In vitro fertilization is Latin for "fertilization under glass" because the fertilization used to take place in a glass lab dish. Today, plastic ones are used.

But what is in vitro fertilization, exactly? IVF—as it is often called—is a remarkable tool to help couples who cannot naturally unite an egg and sperm in the fallopian tubes and/or send an embryo on its merry way into the uterus. A few decades ago, such couples were pretty much out of luck. These days, doctors can often do the "heavy lifting" for them—by retrieving eggs from a woman and sperm from her partner, combining the two in a laboratory dish, then transferring the newly created embryos directly into the woman's uterus for implantation. That's the way it was done way back in 1978 and that's the way it is done now, but the process has improved greatly along with the statistics. How have methods changed over the years? At its inception, IVF was performed without the aid of fertility medications or fancy lab equipment. That is to say, doctors extracted a single ripe egg from the ovary and attempted to fertilize it with sperm. Then, if fertilization occurred, they injected the embryo into the uterus and crossed their fingers in the hope that implantation would occur. (It rarely did.)

Currently, fertility doctors known as *reproductive endocrinologists* ("REs" for short) make use of a family of sophisticated fertility medications to stimulate the development of 4 to 30 eggs as well as to set the stage for healthy implantation by deliberately thickening the uterine lining. They rely on a bag of microscopic tricks to coax the fertilization process along, including intracytoplasmic sperm injection (ICSI), the injection of a single sperm into an egg to jumpstart fertilization, and assisted hatching, the drilling of a teeny hole into the outer shell of the embryo to help it hatch out and continue its essential cell division. They routinely cryopreserve live embryos for use a few months or several years down the road in later cycles. Most importantly, though, doctors hone their treatment plans to make their protocols more effective for a wider variety of couples.

A Peek at the Process

Some of you with a flair for science may know the steps of IVF inside and out. Others may be exploring the process for the very first time (perhaps with a nagging fear that you'll never be able to wrap your head around a science that routinely makes use of procedures with technical, 30-letter names like the previously mentioned *intracytoplasmic sperm injection*). I know I felt that way. Rest assured, you *will* begin to understand the process—and its particular lexicon—more deeply as you read this book and pursue treatment. To get your feet wet, let's begin with the basics.

An IVF cycle usually takes place over the course of a little more than a month. (For a sample calendar, see pages 6–7.) However, your reproductive endocrinologist will certainly need to meet with you well in advance to run necessary tests and develop an appropriate treatment plan befitting both partners. A 25-year-old woman with polycystic ovarian syndrome, for example, will likely require a different cocktail of fertility drugs than a 41-year-old with a diminished egg supply. And dosages vary widely, with some patients requiring four times as much superovulatory medication as others. In addition, many IVFers will require subtler tweaks, such as taking a birth control pill for a month prior to the start of their cycles to improve egg quality. The truth is that no two in-vitro protocols are exactly the same. Nevertheless, all of them follow these six important steps:

Step 1: Suppression and Developing Eggs

Step 2: Retrieving Eggs

Step 3: Developing Embryos

Step 4: Transferring Embryos

Step 5: Preparing the Uterus

Step 6: Pregnancy Test(s)

Although there's a bit of overlap in these steps, each is essential to a successful pregnancy. Now let's take a closer look.

Step 1: Suppression and Developing Eggs

During normal ovulation, women typically release a single egg from their ovaries. During IVF, REs rely on a combination of carefully timed medications to stimulate the development of considerably more. Why? The greater the number of eggs doctors have to work with, the better their chances of creating high-quality embryos that, if all goes well, will develop into bouncing babies.

The first type of medication most IVFers take is called a *gonadotropin-releasing hormone agonist*. (Fear not, you'll probably never have to utter this mouthful.) The majority are prescribed a brand by the name of Lupron. The first shot of Lupron is like a checkered flag signifying the official start of an in-vitro cycle. These daily injections—which typically begin about seven days before a patient's anticipated period—have the important job of "turning off" natural ovulation. Although it may sound counterintuitive to turn off ovulation, it actually makes a lot of sense. Lupron enables REs to control the course of a patient's egg development and prevents unexpected ovulation.

Sample IVF Calendar

Sunday	Monday	Tuesday	Wednesday
Day 1 **Begin Lupron** Suppression	Day 2 Suppression	Day 3 Suppression	Day 4 Suppression
Day 8 **Period** Suppression	Day 9 **Begin Stimulation** Develop Eggs	Day 10 Develop Eggs	Day 11 Develop Eggs
Day 15 Develop Eggs	Day 16 Develop Eggs	Day 17 **HCG Shot** Develop Eggs	Day 18 Develop Eggs
Day 22 Transfer Embryos (Day 3) Prep Uterus	Day 23 OR ⟷ Embryo development continues for 5-day transfers Prep Uterus	Day 24 Transfer Embryos (Day 5) Prep Uterus	Day 25 Prep Uterus
Day 29 Prep Uterus	Day 30 Prep Uterus	Day 31 Prep Uterus	Day 32 Prep Uterus

Thursday	Friday	Saturday
Day 5	**Day 6**	**Day 7**
Suppression	Suppression	Suppression
Day 12	**Day 13**	**Day 14**
Develop Eggs	Develop Eggs	Develop Eggs
Day 19	**Day 20**	**Day 21**
Sperm Sample	Develop Embryos	Develop Embryos
Retrieve Eggs	Prep Uterus	Prep Uterus
Day 26	**Day 27**	**Day 28**
Prep Uterus	Prep Uterus	Prep Uterus
Day 33	**Day 34**	**Day 35** **Prepping continues if pregnant**
	Pregnancy Test	
Prep Uterus	Prep Uterus	Prep Uterus

Yes, Lupron temporarily shuts down ovulation, but it doesn't shut down menstruation. When an IVFer's period arrives, her dosage is reduced and she begins daily injections of one or a combination of two *superovulatory drugs*. Superovulatory drugs are so named because they bring about "super ovulation," a state in which the ovaries "grow" *many* viable eggs as opposed to only one. Brand names include Follistim, Gonal F, Repronex, and Bravelle. Think of them as fertilizer. Over the course of roughly 8 to 12 days, the woman receives daily shots and, with each passing day, her eggs get a little more mature. During this critical phase, doctors keep close tabs on their development with frequent blood tests and sonograms. The blood tests monitor a type of estrogen called *estradiol* (steadily increasing levels are a good sign); the ultrasounds enable REs to see, count, and measure tiny, expanding blisterlike follicles that each contain a developing egg. When the follicles are nearly full size—a mere 15 to 18 millimeters in diameter—the woman is injected with a third medication called *human chorionic gonadotropin,* HCG for short. Administering this special shot is like pushing a button to activate ovulation—only there's a delay. About 40 hours later, the patient's eggs will be released from the ovaries.

Step 2: Retrieving Eggs

HCG shots are precisely timed to enable REs to collect eggs just prior to their peak of maturity—in other words, a few hours *before* ovulation. Say, for example, the shot's given at midnight on Monday. Then, the egg retrieval will be scheduled for Wednesday at noon (or 36 hours later). No ifs, ands, or buts. If this window of opportunity is missed, the cycle will be a bust. During the painless procedure, the patient is sedated with a light anesthesia. As she sleeps, the RE uses an ultrasound probe to visualize both ovaries—now dotted with enlarged follicles filled with ripe-and-ready eggs. Next, a thin needle is inserted through the vagina until it reaches the ovaries. The RE then drains each enlarged follicle, gently sucking the eggs into a special syringe. Time elapsed: about 20 minutes. Moments later, the eggs are transferred to individual lab dishes carefully labeled with the patient's name and she's awakened and provided with a rough count of how many were retrieved. The average number is 5 to 12.

Step 3: Developing Embryos

While the woman is busy undergoing egg retrieval, her partner is equally engaged. He's off in a private room—perhaps leafing through a stack of racy magazines—producing the semen containing the sperm that will be used to fertilize the eggs. Although it may sound challenging to generate a sample under such pressure, most men manage just fine. (And just in case there's a problem, backup sperm has usually been prefrozen.)

As the eggs rest comfortably in nutrient-rich lab dishes, the sperm are washed and tested to help doctors select the best specimens for fertilization. Next, about 50,000 to 100,000 of the heartiest ones are mixed in with each egg. May the best sperm win! In cases where the man's output is less than stellar or seemingly healthy sperm are not penetrating the egg—about 50 percent of the time—doctors rely on intracytoplasmic sperm injection, otherwise known as ICSI. In this now commonplace procedure, a single sperm is injected directly into each egg to shortcut the fertilization process. Both methods are highly successful.

After the eggs and sperm are combined, embryologists use high-powered microscopes to watch for tentative signs of fertilization. Potential embryos start with two teeny cells that divide and divide; within 24 hours they should contain two pronuclei, within 48 hours they should contain at least two cells, and within 72 hours they should contain at least six cells. About 60 to 80 percent of eggs develop into early embryos, but not all of these have the right stuff to be transferred to the uterus. Thus, doctors give each embryo a report card—recording grades of "excellent," "good," "so-so," and "poor" based on the number and the symmetry of their cells. Excellent and good embryos stand the very best chance of continuing to develop into fetuses and then wailing babies.

Step 4: Transferring Embryos

Following the creation of bona fide embryos, REs are charged with the task of delivering them safely to the uterus. This exciting step usually takes place three or five days after egg retrieval. How is this timetable decided? If a couple has a small number of thriving embryos—say two—it makes sense to do the transfer three days after egg retrieval with the thought that they'll thrive better in the natural confines of the uterus rather than in a lab dish. If, however, a couple has a large number of thriving embryos—say 10—it's wiser to let them continue to divide and divide, *then* choose the very best ones to transfer five days after egg retrieval. (Day-three embryos generally have six to eight cells, while five-day embryos have about 100 cells.) Extra-high-quality embryos can be frozen for future cycles.

Another key decision that gets made at this stage is just how many embryos to transfer. The general rule of thumb is two to four. Most practices have strict guidelines based on a woman's age. Younger women get fewer; older women get more. Limiting the number of embryos placed in utero reduces the odds of triplet and quad pregnancies, which are considered high risk.

The good news about an embryo transfer is that it doesn't require anesthesia and is almost always painless. On transfer day, the patient—sometimes giddy with excitement—arrives at her doctor's office and lies on her back with her feet in stirrups. Often, her partner is invited to stand by her side. Often, they're given a microscope snapshot of their developing embryos, magnified thousands of times, to help them visualize their baby- or babies-to-be. The RE then threads a sterile syringe, carefully loaded with their embryos, up through the woman's vagina and gently injects them into her uterus. The process takes mere minutes. Following a half-hour or so of bed rest, patients are usually sent home to take it easy for a few hours or days.

Step 5: Preparing the Uterus

One of the most crucial steps in the IVF timeline is the preparation of the uterine lining. After embryos are injected into the uterus, they float around like minuscule astronauts for a day or two. Then, if all goes well, one or more cozy into the uterine wall for an extended stay. If the endometrial lining is not sufficiently thick and sticky, the embryo (or embryos) won't implant and won't survive. For that reason, REs work hard to ensure it's just right. To achieve this goal, women begin nightly injections (or suppositories) of a medication called *progesterone* the day after their egg retrieval. This viscous natural hormone serves to build up the uterine lining to make it extra receptive to incoming embryos. Progesterone treatment continues until the first pregnancy test and well beyond if a pregnancy is established.

Step 6: Pregnancy Test(s)
If IVF is a roller coaster ride, this final stretch is the climactic loop-to-loop. Patients listen to their bodies with pin-drop intensity—one day they "know" they're pregnant, the next day they "know" they're not. The truth is, at this stage, it's impossible for even the most body-conscious women to tell. Doctors, however, *can* diagnose an early, early pregnancy with a simple blood test. The first one takes place about 10 to 14 days after the embryo transfer. If HCG—a hormone produced by an implanted embryo—is detected, that's an auspicious sign. And if the HCG level continues to double every couple days, that means a baby-to-be is likely developing. That being said, REs remain cautiously optimistic, testing and retesting patients a number of times over the course of several weeks until they're able to detect a fetal heartbeat—or two or three—at about week seven. That gentle thrumming signifies the close of a successful in-vitro cycle and the happy couple graduates to an OB/GYN.

That's it—the six basic steps of in vitro fertilization. Don't despair if you're still a bit fuzzy on the particulars. I guarantee they'll come into sharper focus as you read on. (In fact, Chapters 8 and 9 provide a detailed description of every aspect of the process.) In the meantime, let's turn our attention to a few noteworthy statistics.

Interpreting IVF Statistics

IVF numbers, which can be sliced and diced a zillion different ways, can get pretty overwhelming. For that reason, it's probably wise to stick to the must-know statistics. A good place to start is with a look at the conditions that cause couples to seek out in vitro in the first place.

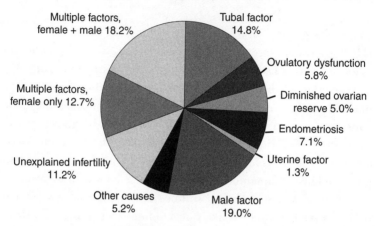

Reasons People Pursue IVF
From the CDC ART Report, 2001

Multiple factors, female + male 18.2%

Tubal factor 14.8%

Ovulatory dysfunction 5.8%

Diminished ovarian reserve 5.0%

Multiple factors, female only 12.7%

Endometriosis 7.1%

Uterine factor 1.3%

Unexplained infertility 11.2%

Other causes 5.2%

Male factor 19.0%

* Total does not equal 100% due to rounding

Do you see yourself reflected in a piece of this pie chart? Perhaps you've been recently diagnosed with a blocked tube or have just been referred to a fertility center because your OB/GYN suspects you may have polycystic ovarian syndrome. Maybe your doctor can't quite pinpoint the source of your problems and you fall into the 11.2 percent of couples with unexplained causes. Lily, a 39-year-old writer and mom of a daughter born via IVF, remembers finding a chart like this comforting. "I located myself and my husband among the sizable group with both female *and* male factors and it made me feel better. It gave us some confidence to find that we were part of a club we jokingly began to refer to as 'the infertility overachievers.'" That's right, you're not alone: People struggling with each of these issues have found effective treatment with IVF. Here's a quick 101 on these conditions and how IVF can help:

❧ **Tubal Factors:** (14.8 percent) Chronic infections, sometimes due to undetected sexually transmitted diseases, can cause blockages of the fallopian tubes—the all-important location where fertilization takes place. That means sperm and eggs cannot meet and "mate." IVF bypasses the problem by whisking embryos directly to the uterus.

❧ **Ovulatory Dysfunction:** (5.8 percent) Because of a surplus or deficit of key hormones, ovaries can malfunction sporadically or stop working altogether. This category includes women with polycystic ovarian syndrome whose ovaries form cysts instead of mature eggs due to a high influx of luteinizing hormone. The special medications and monitoring used during IVF help these women's bodies yield healthy eggs.

❧ **Diminished Ovarian Reserve:** (5.0 percent) Ovaries are like banks filled with eggs. Although each woman's biological clock ticks at a different speed, everyone's stockpile gets diminished and damaged over time. For this reason, the problem is especially common in women 37 and above. The fertility medications used during IVF help the ovaries develop more mature eggs, dramatically increasing the chances of successful fertilization.

❧ **Endometriosis:** (7.1 percent) When the endometrial lining sheds each month, bits of it sometimes implant and continue to grow—and grow—outside the uterus. Endometriosis on the ovaries or fallopian tubes can cause damage that keeps them from doing their essential jobs. As with blocked tubes, IVF circumvents the problem by delivering the embryos directly to the uterus.

❧ **Uterine Factors:** (1.3 percent) Occasionally, a structural or functional issue related to the uterus stands in the way of healthy implantation. IVF sometimes solves the problem by getting embryos to their intended destination *and* creating a receptive uterine lining.

୬ **Male Factor:** (19.0 percent) Although male factor accounts for 40 percent of all infertility, some people are still not aware that it can be effectively treated with IVF. This category includes men with low-count or poor-quality sperm. It also includes those with no detectable sperm count at all, due to blocked or missing transport tubes. In such cases, doctors can often extract the sperm from a man's testicles via a fine needle, then use ICSI—the process of injecting a single sperm into an egg—to bring about fertilization.

୬ **Other Causes:** (5.2 percent) This catch-all category includes women with immune and antibody disorders, chromosomal abnormalities, and a history of chemotherapy or serious illness that have affected their ability to reproduce. IVF can sometimes come to the rescue by helping healthy embryos implant in the uterus.

୬ **Unexplained Causes:** (11.2 percent) Try as they might, doctors are sometimes unable to determine the cause of a couple's infertility. As their diagnostic tools become more sophisticated, however, this category will likely shrink and possibly vanish altogether. For now, IVF is a good bet because it can override a host of undetected issues.

୬ **Multiple Factors, Female:** (12.7 percent) Because women have more bells and whistles in their reproductive system than men, it is not uncommon for them to have two—or three—fertility issues at once, such as endometriosis *and* diminished ovarian reserve. In many cases, IVF enables doctors to tackle multiple problems in one fell swoop.

୬ **Multiple Factors, Female and Male:** (18.2 percent) Unfortunately, a woman's fertility problem does not preclude her partner having one, too. IVF is a good way to address both issues in a single treatment.

Now, let's explore the per-cycle birth rates by diagnosis:

Per-Cycle Birth Rates by Diagnosis
Using Fresh, Nondonor Eggs
From the CDC ART Report, 2001

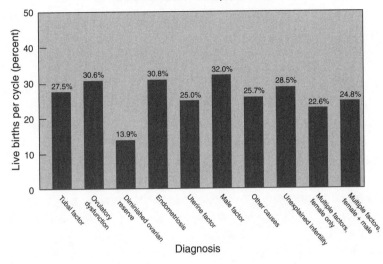

For those of you thinking the statistics on this chart are not quite as rosy as you'd hoped, let me offer a few encouraging words. First, these numbers are based on live births reported by hundreds of in-vitro clinics. It takes three years to collect all the data. During that period, science marches on and REs hone their craft. My point? The odds of achieving IVF success today are better than they were even three years ago. (In fact, some programs report an increase of 5 percent or more annually!) Second, because success rates vary widely from practice to practice, you can dramatically increase your chances of achieving a healthy pregnancy by seeking out an experienced top-tier clinic with statistics *well above* the national average represented here. As mentioned earlier, the best ones report per-cycle birth rates close to 50 percent! (Important tips for locating a great practice are covered in Chapter 6.)

Finally, and most importantly, because these numbers are drawn from IVFers who remain anonymous, there's no way to track the final outcome of women who undergo the process more than once. There's comfort in the fact that this bar graph does not reflect the "ultimate" success rates of couples who bring home babies following a second, third, or even fourth cycle. If it did, these statistics would increase by leaps and bounds. In fact, some experts estimate the percentage of IVFers who achieve their goal of parenthood with multiple tries to be as high as 75 percent!

Why are multiple tries so important? In some ways, in vitro is like a coin toss. Let's say you call "heads." If you don't get it on your first toss, the simple act of tossing a second and third time will certainly increase your chances of doing so. Same goes for IVF. If your first cycle doesn't succeed, there's a good chance the second or third will. But there's another reason the odds increase with fresh tries. They give doctors an opportunity to learn from their mistakes. REs carefully evaluate every failed cycle in an attempt to figure out how each protocol can be improved. This helps stack the cards in an IVFer's favor. Should the patient begin her cycle with the birth control pill? Should the superovulatory medication be switched to another brand? Was the dosage too low or too high? Even little tweaks to a treatment plan can make a big difference.

No question, we'd all like IVF to work the first time around, but sometimes it doesn't. Therefore, it's important to try to think of it as a process rather than a quick fix. Says Judy, a 33-year-old art director: "When my first stab at IVF failed I was really depressed. I didn't know if I had the stamina to do it again, but my doctor helped convince me that I had a good shot with a different type of medication. It took a total of three cycles, which costs more than I would like, but it was totally worth it. I have my precious son."

Next, let's look at the ages of women who pursue IVF, using their own eggs. As you can see from the graph on page 17, the data take the shape of a classic bell curve. Although a handful of women under 24 and over 44 pursue IVF, the vast majority are between the ages of 30 and 40. (It's important to note, however, that the sizable pool of women who use donor eggs—and who tend to be 40 or more—are not re-

Ages of Women Who Do IVF Using Fresh, Nondonor Eggs
From the CDC ART Report, 2001

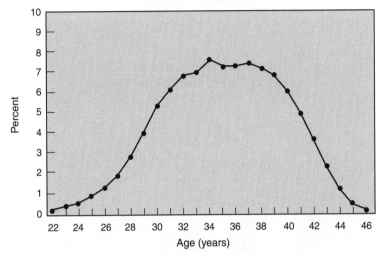

flected here.) Why is IVF mostly for the over-30 set? The simple answer is that many of us choose to postpone motherhood. To start with, we're getting married older. In the 1950s the average age of a bride was 20, today it's 25. Let's face it, though, a lot of us don't meet Mr. Right until we're deep into our thirties or forties. (And some are still looking!) Then there's that little thing called a job. Meaningful work is fulfilling and certainly essential for paying your bills and saving for the future. Thus, it's quite common for women to put off starting a family until they're on track with a career and have some cash socked away.

Makes a lot of sense, right? The only downside is that many of us are not as fertile as we were at 22—the age some of our mothers were when they had us. As we mature, egg quality slowly declines and issues such as fibroids or tubal obstructions can become more serious. As a result, a thirty-something who's decided the time is finally right to have a baby may find herself face to face with a fertility roadblock. That was certainly true for me. My ducks were finally in a row: I had a great marriage, a solid career, a grown-up apartment in Manhattan with a pepper grinder—even a little money tucked away. The only glitch was that I couldn't get pregnant, no matter how hard I tried. It soon became clear that IVF was the key.

Last, but not least, let's take a look at IVF success rates by age:

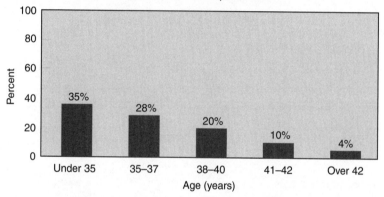

Per-Cycle Birth Rates By Age Using Fresh, Nondonor Eggs
From the CDC ART Report, 2001

Age is the single most important predictor of IVF success. When a woman passes 28, her fertility starts to subtly slide, with a dip around 35 and a steeper decline after 40. Why? Over the years, hormonal changes can cause the intricate symphony of monthly ovulation to become a little—or a lot—out of tune. Conditions such as fibroids, endometriosis, or tubal blockages may get worse. Ovaries contain fewer eggs, as a hundred or so vanish each month following ovulation. As we get older, some eggs remain perfectly healthy, while others sustain microscopic damage that will inhibit them from fertilizing or implanting. "Eggs age," states Dr. Lawrence Werlin, a renowned RE at Coastal Fertility Medical Center in Irvine, California. "Over time, some simply wear out like the heart muscle or even a pair of gloves."

Yes, age is significant, but it's not everything. Fact: Millions and millions of women well beyond their "peak" of fertility bring home babies. In fact, at the moment I have four very pregnant girlfriends—ages 40, 41, 42, and 43! Jeanie, a 35-year-old business manager gearing up for her first round of IVF, puts it well: "A relative of mine gently told me to prepare to have trouble getting pregnant since I'd just turned 35. It seems she'd read some article on the topic in a major magazine. That upset me a lot at first. Then I came to realize that reaching 35 wasn't like jumping off a diving board into a pool of infertility. In fact, my issue—polycystic ovaries—had been diagnosed in my early twenties. If my ability to have a baby was declining, it was declining slowly. Maybe it wouldn't be quite as easy to get pregnant, but it was still very probable, especially with the help of a fertility doctor."

Fertility Fact: In 1923, the female hormone estrogen was discovered. Scientists found progesterone in 1929.

OK, the bad news is that IVF is not a sure thing for anyone. The good news is that it is a very effective treatment for women at a variety of ages and stages of life. And for those who simply can't get pregnant with their own eggs, donor ova—eggs harvested from another woman—offer the remarkable opportunity to nurture a baby in utero. Granted, it's a serious decision to carry a child that is genetically linked to your partner but not to you. It isn't for everyone. However, for the thousands of couples who pursue it, the odds of having a healthy baby are extremely high, rivaling the success rates of women in their twenties. (We will spend much more time on that important topic in Chapter 7.)

A Final Word on Statistics

Fact: You are *not* a statistic.

So the question on the tip of your tongue is probably, *Why are you showing me all these statistics and then telling me I'm not one?* Statistics are percentages and pie charts and black-and-white numbers. You are a person who wants to have a baby. Consider the story of Yvette, a 42-year-old nurse. She recalls her own struggle with the numbers game:

"Because of my job, I was used to looking at lab results—so I knew that I was far from an ideal candidate for IVF. My FSH [follicle-stimulating hormone] was a bit too high, so was my estradiol. Yes, I knew the score, but I still had a strong feeling that in vitro could work for me. So I made an appointment at a really good practice, sat down, and had a frank discussion with the RE. He didn't make me any promises, of course, but agreed it was certainly worth trying. Lo and behold, it took just one cycle to get pregnant with Jack Jr. I'm really, really glad I went with my gut."

I remember how I felt on the brink of IVF, my optimism rising and falling with each new "fact" I gleaned—many from some fairly questionable sources. After a while my head was spinning, but I was pretty paralyzed. Then I realized that I couldn't have "all of the facts" until I met with my doctor. And even then, I would not be a carbon copy of any other woman in his practice—even if I looked similar on paper. While it's essential to get a handle on numbers and be realistic about your chances for success, it's also important to know that you are unique. Your fertility profile is unique, your body is unique, and your circumstances are unique.

So take a deep breath and know you are not a dot on a graph. There is a much bigger picture to take into account, including your heredity, hormone levels, personal ovarian reserve, uterine lining, partner's semen analysis, and, to some degree, your determination. Infertility is not a one-size-fits-all diagnosis. Fact: Thanks to IVF, tens of thousands of women in their twenties, thirties, and forties have fulfilled their dreams of motherhood. Certainly, your RE will be able to give you a better sense of your odds for succeeding after examining you and running key tests. Listen closely, but ask questions. Be practical, but hopeful. And, most importantly, do not discount your own instincts. After all, no one knows your body better than you.

Chapter 2

Getting a Fix
on Your Infertility

ॐ

The Courage to Get Answers

Do these five stages of infertility sound familiar?

1. You decide you want a baby, deep-six the birth control, and start having carefree sex.

2. Carefree sex isn't working quickly enough so you begin timing your lovemaking sessions to loosely correspond with ovulation. You tell yourself you're not worried.

3. Still no luck, so you head to the drugstore and purchase an ovulation predictor to help get a better fix on your window of opportunity. Now you mean business!

4. The ovulation kit hasn't done the trick yet, but you decide to give it a few more tries. Your mood rises and falls with your monthly menstrual cycle. When your period arrives you burst into tears.

5. OK, now you're upset. You summon your courage and take the first tentative steps toward finding out what's really going on.

Chances are you've had firsthand experience with each one of these stages. Chances are, too, that you're confused and more than a little frustrated. That was certainly the case for Sarah. After this 29-year-old paralegal tied the knot, she and her husband wanted kids right away. And, like most of us, she assumed getting pregnant would be a snap. "My little sister was so fertile. It was the family joke that her husband would just look at her, then—Zap!—she'd be pregnant. She was 27 and already had three kids! Naturally, I thought the same rule would apply to me. But a whole year passed without a pregnancy, whether I timed intercourse or stood on my head. After a while, I got depressed, I got tired."

I remember that frame of mind well. Dealing with month after month of failed conception can sap the strength of even the heartiest individuals. But that doesn't mean you should give up. Help is on the way in the form of this chapter. In the pages that follow, I'll list the "red flags" that signify it's time to seek out a specialist. In addition, I'll outline what to expect during a standard fertility work-up, including a roundup of the most popular tools used to diagnose problems and decide if IVF is a possible solution. No question, it takes courage to find out what's wrong. But determining what's amiss is the first stepping-stone on the path to your baby. So read on.

The Definition of Infertility

It is estimated that more than six million American women are affected by infertility, which translates to about 1 in 10 of the childbearing population. Look around you: Many of the folks you see at the office or the deli or the yoga studio are having trouble, too. This year, one million of them will seek specialized medical treatment. And, of this group, a few hundred thousand will seriously consider IVF.

But what does "affected by infertility" mean exactly? Strictly speaking, any couple who tries unsuccessfully to have a baby for one year is considered to have some level of infertility. Does that mean there is no chance they will ever conceive naturally? Of course not. It does mean, however, that they should probably consult an experienced doctor to find out what can be done to maximize their chances. Even if they are in their early twenties. Even if they've had a baby in the past. Fertility-compromising issues, such as male factor or decreased ovarian reserve, have a tendency to sneak up on unsuspecting individuals and reduce their chances of conceiving. Fertility exists on a continuum, with some couples having everything in place—quality cervical mucus, balanced hormones, open tubes, high sperm count—to speed the process along, while others are forced to contend with minor to major stumbling blocks.

To get a fix on infertility, let's take a look at the six factors that should be present to achieve a natural pregnancy:

1. Sexual intercourse near the time of ovulation.

2. The release of a healthy, mature egg from the ovaries.

3. An ample supply of strong, well-formed sperm deposited in the upper vagina, leading to the cervical canal.

4. Thin, nutrient-rich cervical mucus (to help sperm make its way to the fallopian tubes).

5. Open, disease-free fallopian tubes (where the sperm and egg can meet and "mate").

6. A healthy uterus with a thick endometrial lining (which enables a developing embryo to take hold).

If any one of these six factors is compromised, the odds of getting pregnant are significantly decreased. But even for those with "normal" fertility, the reproductive drama is pretty intense. In fact, if conception were a movie it would resemble a kick-butt, action-adventure flick far more than a tender romance. Why? Although sperm are required to travel a mere four inches from the vagina to the fallopian tubes, that's a Herculean feat when you consider their size—500 times smaller than a grain of sand! That means their grueling journey is the equivalent of a human being swimming the English Channel more than 1,000 times! In addition, sperm have to navigate the treacherous terrain of the cervical canal. If the mucus there is too thick, they won't be able to swim through it. If a bit of K-Y Jelly was used during sex, its toxic presence could put the kibosh on half of them. In the end, only a small fraction of the millions of sperm will survive the grueling pilgrimage.

But let's not forget the egg. Its role is equally dramatic. Each month, roughly one hundred race to ripen. But only one (occasionally two) wins the competition and actually gets released from the ovaries. The rest simply dissolve. During ovulation, the fingerlike fimbriae at the end of the fallopian tube gently suck the lead egg off the ovary and guide it *inside* one of the tubes. There—if the timing is just right—a few hundred of the heartiest sperm will be on hand for the primitive mating ritual. Of them, just one (if any) has the right stuff to beat the others to the punch and penetrate the egg—nearly 600 times its size! If that happens, the two fuse together to form an early embryo. But don't roll the credits yet. Now it's the embryo's turn to take a four- to five-day journey all the way to the uterus, dividing and dividing en route. *If* it gets there and *if* the endometrial lining is sufficiently thick, then, and only then, does that embryo have a decent shot of implanting in the uterine wall and developing into a full-fledged fetus. Time elapsed: about seven days.

Sound treacherous and exciting and exhausting and remarkable? It is. Achieving a healthy pregnancy is also one of the most common events in the world, occurring more than four million times annually in the United States alone. When I used to get overwhelmed with all the hurdles my body needed to jump through to get me pregnant, I reminded myself that conception is truly miraculous for *everyone.* And for those of us with small or sizable "glitches" in our reproductive systems, doctors are often able to step in and right what's wrong—with medications, surgeries, and, yes, IVF. In fact it's estimated that 80 percent of all couples who seek treatment for infertility manage to achieve healthy pregnancies! But doctors can't help us until we help ourselves by taking the necessary steps to figure out what's wrong.

Going to the Doctor

You may not love going to the doctor. But try to get used to it. The IVF process—and the road leading up to it—requires that we put our fears aside and be patient. To figure out whether in vitro makes sense for you, it's essential that both you and your partner have, at the very least, a basic fertility work-up. But even a "basic" work-up can be pretty intensive. By the time you're through, summer may have turned to fall. And you may have read every magazine in your physician's waiting room, right down to the tattered copy of *Quarter Horse Monthly*. (Who put that there anyway?)

During that time frame, some of you will get by with just a few tests while others will feel like they're sampling everything on the poke-and-prod menu. But it's wise to persevere. The more your doctor knows, the better he or she can address your problem. It's also wise for you to have a general understanding of what to expect. This way, when you hear, "Let's check your prolactic level or do a clomiphene challenge or try a hysterosalpingogram," you'll be armed with some notion of what the heck your physician is talking about. And the fact is most of these tests aren't nearly as bad as they sound.

Remember, too, that each one of them brings you closer to your goal. When your arm is sore from an umpteenth stick, when you're awaiting a laparoscopy, when your partner traipses, yet again, to the urologist—remember that this is about having a child. In vitro, with its battery of tests, can seem absurdly scientific and labor-intensive. But when it works, the result is something heartwarmingly old-fashioned: a gurgling, squirming baby. So try to bear with the pokes and prods. In my own experience, nothing hurt more than the pain of giving in to fear and doing nothing. What are the criteria for getting things checked out?

• If you've tried to have a baby for an entire year.

• If you've had irregular periods.

• If you've had two or more miscarriages.

• If you're closing in on 40.

Sometimes basic fertility work-ups are done by your own gynecologist and sometimes by a reproductive endocrinologist ("RE") or, in your partner's case, a urologist. Either way, this series of tests is often covered, at least partially, by insurance, so make sure to check your policy. Who should conduct your work-up? If your current gynecologist seems dismissive, uninterested, or simply lacking in expertise— which may well be the case—it's time to graduate to a specialist.

Fertility Fact: Only 21 percent of infertile women seek medical care to determine the cause of their infertility and/or treat it.

After failing to conceive for two years, I had an inkling I should move on the day my doctor advised me simply "to keep trying." That answer wasn't going to cut it anymore. When your instincts tell you to seek an expert opinion, ask your gynecologist to provide a referral to a great RE. Stress the word *great*. After all, the right doctor can make all the difference. (For tips on choosing a great practice, see Chapter 6.)

The Basic
Fertility Work-up for You

If you're like me, you probably hate the multipage form that greets you whenever you visit a new doctor. Well, in the case of infertility it isn't just busywork. This paperwork has a purpose. Take the necessary time to fill in all of the information to the best of your knowledge. It's important to your diagnosis. And tell the truth. We all have a few skeletons in our closets. Perhaps you experienced a bout of chlamydia or contracted herpes years ago, a reminder of an old boyfriend you'd just as soon forget. As uncomfortable as such memories are, they're essential pieces to your fertility puzzle. So brush off your embarrassment and be prepared to be painfully honest.

Here's what your doctor should cover before beginning your work-up:

ॐ **Your Period:** Ahhh, those beloved menstrual queries: At what age did your period begin? Are you regular? Is your flow light or heavy? Does your PMS rate a 1 or 10 on the Richter scale? This may seem like yada-yada-yada stuff, but it often provides important clues to a woman's infertility.

ॐ **Your Ovulation Schedule:** If you've had trouble getting pregnant, chances are you're already a pro at charting your monthly basal body temperature or using an ovulation predictor to determine your window of fertility. If you noticed that your temperature was elevated mid-cycle or you saw that telltale line on the predictor stick—good news!—you are probably ovulating. Be sure to share this key "intelligence" with your doctor.

ॐ **Health Problems and Surgeries:** Were you ever diagnosed with a thyroid condition? A blood-clotting disorder? A sexually transmitted disease? Did you have an ovary removed because of a cyst? Rupture your appendix in the sixth grade? Have a mom who took DES? Better to err on the side of mentioning *everything*. In the process of turning over every stone, you may uncover a significant factor.

ॐ **Medications:** Put your cards on the table: Do you take an antidepressant? A drug for herpes? An herbal concoction purchased in Chinatown to promote fertility? Americans rely on an array of prescribed, over-the-counter, and holistic drugs to address large and small concerns. Some of them can reduce your ability to conceive.

❧ **Sexual History:** It's critical that you're extremely frank about your sexual history, including pregnancies, miscarriages, abortions, and sexually transmitted diseases. Remember, doctors are professionals and it's unlikely you're telling them something they haven't heard before.

❧ **Sexual Patterns:** How often do you have sex? What types of birth control have you used in the past? (Some IUDs, for example, can cause infertility.) Do you make use of K-Y Jelly? Discontinuing the use of little things like lubricants can actually make a big difference.

❧ **Lifestyle Patterns:** Do you smoke? Drink excessively? Frequently use marijuana or cocaine? Are you struggling with an eating disorder? Yes, we all blanch at such questions, but it's imperative that you answer them and, if need be, take steps to get such problems under control. In addition, overexercising to the point of missing periods can suppress monthly ovulation—and with it your chances of conceiving.

No one shouts, *Hooray, it's time to put my feet in stirrups for my gyno exam!* but such checkups are a necessary evil. And, thankfully, they last only a few minutes. Heather, a 32-year-old speech pathologist, admits to being a card-carrying squeamish type: "I made and canceled about three appointments. Finally, I just went—sweaty palms and all. And you know what? The exam wasn't nearly as bad as I'd built it up to be." Reality seldom competes with an overactive imagination. So try your best to relax, but don't beat yourself up if you're a bit tense. Doctors are used to it.

Make sure your physician gives you a complete pelvic exam, checking your vaginal canal for growths and performing a pap smear (to rule out cervical cancer). He or she should culture your cervical mucus to screen it for infections such as gonorrhea or chlamydia, then feel your thyroid gland for signs of enlargement. (Both over- and underactive thyroid conditions can render you less fertile.) In addition, your breasts should be examined and your nipples squeezed to see if any milk is expressed. Milk production is associated with the overproduction of a hormone called *prolactin*—also present in nursing moms—which can send a message to your body to stop ovulating. Next, as odd as it may sound, your face and groin should be checked for excessive hair, which can point to polycystic ovarian syndrome. Finally, your doctor should perform an ultrasound to get a first look at your reproductive organs, including the size and shape of your uterus. If he or she sees signs of scarring, polyps, endometriosis, or blockages, expect to graduate to a higher-tech evaluation. (See page 34 for more information.)

Testing, Testing

After your consultation and physical exam, prepare for at least a few more tests, some of which may seem a bit kooky. Rest assured, they're not. Your doctor may order a Postcoital Test, for example. This routine exam actually requires you to have sex with your partner—at home, fortunately—then show up at your doctor's office several hours later to have your mucus swabbed and viewed under a microscope. If a good number of his swimmers are still alive and kicking, that means your cervical mucus and his sperm are pretty compatible. Ready for another wacky one? How about the Hamster–Sperm Penetration Test, which—you guessed it!—involves a hamster, or at least its tiny eggs. If your partner's sperm can penetrate hamster eggs, it bodes well that they'll be able to penetrate your eggs, too. (Don't worry, the two species cannot spawn offspring.) Exactly how many tests will you need? That depends on how long it takes to pinpoint your problem. At the very least, everyone should be sure to get a Day-Three FSH Test. (For information on others, see the box on page 32.)

Fertility Fact: The Greek word *hormo*, from which we get "hormone," means to "set in motion, spur on, or excite."

The All-Important
Day-Three FSH Test

First, let's take a quick look at the family of hormones that are essential to conception.

Portrait of a Menstrual Cycle

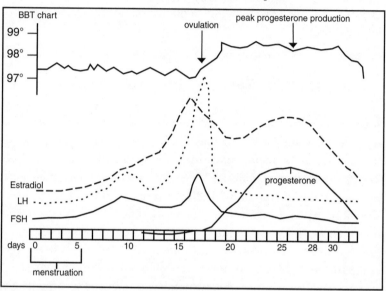

Just after ovulation, your temperature rises a half to a full degree and remains elevated until just before your period. Every month, too, key hormones rise and fall in a carefully orchestrated symphony of fertility. As you can see on the chart above, Follicle-Stimulating Hormone (FSH) and Luteinizing Hormone (LH) begin to ramp up at the start of your period, spiking around ovulation time, then steeply falling right after it. That's because the presence of FSH and LH in your blood actually stimulates your eggs to mature. When the lead egg is released, their work is done. Estradiol (a type of estrogen) also nurtures egg development, but it has a second job as well. Along with progesterone, it stimulates the buildup of the uterine lining, making it thick and sticky so that an incoming embryo can take hold and develop there. For that reason, estradiol has a second influx in the latter half of your cycle. And progesterone doesn't even get started until after ovulation, peaking about day 25, then falling just before menstruation (that is, unless you are pregnant and its services are still required). If the level of any of these hormones is off, it's a strong indication that something is amiss. For that reason, doctors like to keep close tabs on them.

One of the ways they do this is with a Day-Three FSH Test, so called because it measures your FSH on the third day of your period. This simple blood test is perhaps the single most important diagnostic tool an RE has—especially for those 37 or older. Why? As mentioned earlier, ovaries are like personal banks that store and dispense our eggs each month. Although only 400 or so lead eggs get released from our ovaries during our fertile years, another 300,000 plus will get "used up" as they race to ripen during approximately 400 ovulations. Additionally, thousands of other eggs will sustain invisible damage that will inhibit them from developing and implanting. Although every woman is on a different schedule, as menopause draws near, the supply of "good" eggs diminishes. And unfortunately, unlike a man's sperm (which get replenished every 100 days), there is no way to make more. A Day-Three FSH Test helps your doctor assess the status of your ovarian reserve—a fancy way of saying the quantity and quality of the eggs that remain.

How does it work? Your doctor draws blood on day 3 of your menstrual cycle, sends it to the lab, then gets an FSH reading. As you can see from the chart on page 30, your FSH level should be relatively low at that point. Doctors *want* to see a low number there as a high number often signifies a problem. Huh? What I'm saying may sound a bit confusing since I just reported a few paragraphs ago that an influx of FSH actually *helps* to mature the eggs. That's true, but as women age and approach menopause, their general FSH level actually increases to compensate for fewer, older eggs. A gas-pedal-of-a-car analogy is often used to explain this phenomenon. If you have to bear down hard on the gas pedal just to get your car going, it's likely there's a problem with the car. The same holds for a woman's body. If FSH is floored, even on day 3 when its "muscle" isn't yet needed for egg development, chances are there's an issue with her ovarian reserve.

So what numbers are doctors looking for? Since the test is not standardized, it depends on the lab your blood work gets sent to. For some, less than 10 mIU/ml (milli-International Units per milliliter) is considered normal; for others, it's less than 20 mIU/ml. Thus, it's essential that your doctor interpret the results for you before you jump to any conclusions. Like many other fertility factors, FSH levels exist on a continuum, with any given woman having a great, good, so-so, or poor reading. Where do you fall on that spectrum? Although there are no absolutes, it's wise to have a frank discussion with your physician concerning this important question. Be a realist, but remember—It takes only one good egg to make a baby. If your doctor suspects a problem, he or she may try to get a more detailed portrait of your ovarian reserve by taking a look at some other key hormone levels, including estradiol and progesterone. (For more information, see the box below.)

More Tests for Her

Here's a roundup of other tests that your doctor may want you to take:

Estradiol Test: As with FSH, an elevated estradiol level can also signify problems with your eggs. This blood test is also conducted on day 3, often in tandem with the FSH test. A reading of less than 50 pg/ml (pictograms per milliliter) is considered normal, while a reading above 75 pg/ml is an indication of reduced ovarian reserve.

Luteinizing Hormone (LH) Test: Because LH triggers ovulation, it's imperative to have an adequate level. If you've used a drugstore ovulation kit in the past and seen that telltale line—great! That's a strong indicator that your body is making LH. That being said, *too* much LH can be problematic and is often associated with polycystic ovarian syndrome.

Clomiphene Citrate Challenge: This multistep test provides a more detailed snapshot of your ovarian reserve than a standard FSH test. In addition, it offers clues as to how your ovaries will respond to superovulatory drugs. First, FSH and estradiol levels are measured on day 3 of your menstrual cycle, then clomiphene citrate pills are taken on days 5 to 9. Finally, FSH is measured again on day 10. Elevated day-3 or day-10 FSH (as well as day-3 estradiol) are all strong indications of reduced ovarian reserve.

Progesterone Test: This blood test measures your progesterone level one week before your period. Since progesterone rises following ovulation, an elevated level at this juncture is a strong sign that ovulation is occurring.

Prolactin Test: Excess prolactin can affect fertility because it tricks the body into thinking it's pregnant, which means you won't ovulate and/or build up a sufficient endometrial lining. This simple blood test can be done during any day of the cycle.

Thyroid-Stimulating Hormone Test: Because the thyroid gland plays a key role in maintaining hormonal balance, it sometimes stands in the way of healthy pregnancies. Thyroid conditions are prevalent among women in their thirties and forties. In fact, a recent study asserts that as many as 13 million Americans have a thyroid-related health problem and don't even know it! This blood test will tell if you fall into that category. The good news is that these conditions are easily treatable.

Total Testosterone and Dehydroepiandrosterone Sulfate Tests: Yes, women have testosterone, too! A surplus of either of these "male" hormones can cause acne, excessive body hair, irregular periods, and fertility issues. Chances are you don't have a problem, but this quick blood test will tell you for sure.

Postcoital Test: Have you heard the one about the man's sperm that was allergic to his wife's cervical mucus? No, this isn't the setup for a corny one-liner. Occasionally, sperm quality is compromised by the chemical makeup of a woman's cervical mucus. This test involves having sex with your partner at home around ovulation time, then showing up at your doctor's office 2 to 12 hours later. There, a sample of your mucus gets swabbed and viewed under a microscope. Three or more sperm still moving are a "thumbs up" that your mucus and his sperm are a good match.

More Tests for Her *(continued on next page)*

More Tests for Her *(continued)*

Endometrial Biopsy: The buildup of the endometrial lining is essential to a healthy pregnancy—without it, an embryo won't be able to stick and stay. This test, which is usually given on day 21 of your cycle, entails threading a thin, needlelike instrument up into the uterus to gather a tiny sample of tissue. The sample is then tested to see if it's thick and sticky enough to support implantation.

Immune Testing: There is much controversy about the usefulness of immune testing to uncover possible roadblocks to successful implantation and pregnancies. Although the American Society of Reproductive Medicine does not yet endorse such screening, some experts are firm believers that locating and addressing immunologic issues—such as antibody disorders—hold the key to fertility for a minority of couples.

Karyotyping: In cases of multiple miscarriage, doctors will sometimes order an analysis of the chromosomes to determine if any abnormalities are present that may be triggering the problem.

Taking a Look at the Reproductive Organs

Unfortunately, blood tests alone are usually not enough to get a definitive take on your infertility. Even if doctors uncover a hormonal or egg-related factor, such as high FSH, that "Aha!" doesn't rule out the presence of a structural factor, too. For that reason, a woman's reproductive organs are often examined to make sure they're in good working order. The following are the three most popular diagnostic tools used for this purpose.

Hysterosalpingogram (HSG Test)

What a name! In the beginning, I stumbled over the word *hysterosalpingogram* every time I attempted to say it. After a while, I wised up and began referring to it by its nickname: the HSG Test. The purpose of this X-ray procedure, usually performed by a radiologist, is to get an initial read on the condition of your fallopian tubes and uterus. As with a number of tests related to infertility, it's typically scheduled for

---

Fertility Fact: A girl baby is born with about seven million eggs, but by the time she reaches puberty there are only about 700,000 left.

---

the first half of your menstrual cycle, after your period but prior to ovulation. This timetable increases the doctor's visibility but reduces the chance, however minimal, that you'll be pregnant during the procedure. How does it work? As you lie on your back with your feet in stirrups, a catheter is inserted through your cervix and into your uterus. Then a contrast dye is injected. If the dye flies through your uterus and tubes into your abdominal cavity, that's a good sign: It means your tubes are open. If it doesn't, there's likely a blockage. A series of X-rays are taken for documentation.

In addition to diagnosing blockages, the HSG Test can turn up a host of other abnormalities—such as fibroids and scar tissue—which show up as suspicious, shadowy patches on the X-rays. Yes, this test can cause minor cramping, but, thankfully, it's brief—often taking less time than a trip to the dentist. And here's more good news: Occasionally, the mere act of forcing the dye through your tubes can dislodge pesky debris, clearing the way for natural pregnancy. If your doctor suspects a problem, however, your next step will likely be a laparoscopy.

Laparoscopy

When doctors want to take a closer look at or treat problems related to the ovaries, fallopian tubes, and outer wall of the uterus, they often opt for laparoscopy. Unlike the HSG Test, this surgical procedure is usually performed at a hospital and requires anesthesia. Beforehand, you'll be instructed not to eat or drink anything after 12 midnight and should be given antibiotics to safeguard against infection. You'll also be required to sign a release form outlining a number of unpleasant complications that may arise. Although many of them sound pretty scary, know that this procedure is performed thousands of times each year and is actually very safe.

Know, too, that it's one of the best ways to get to the bottom of your fertility problem. Here's how it works. While you are asleep, a lighted telescopelike instrument called a *laparoscope*—about twice as long as a fountain pen—is inserted through a tiny incision just below your navel. After that, carbon dioxide is pumped into the pelvis to separate the organs and make them easier to see. Next, the doctor will play detective by searching each of them for signs of endometriosis, fibroids, polyps, and the like. Then, in many cases, he or she will attempt to remove the offending "items" on the spot with the aid of delicate tools or laser surgery. The entire process takes thirty minutes to two hours, depending on what needs to be done.

When the process is over, you'll be sent home to take it easy for a couple days. Expect to feel wiped out and bloated from the gas, which takes a while to work its way out of your system. "I remember feeling like a beach ball," reports Carla, a 32-year-old homemaker. "I also remember feeling a mix of emotions. It was upsetting to learn that I had a severely blocked tube, which could not be corrected through surgery. But I was also happy that we *finally, finally* figured out what the problem was. Knowing that IVF was the logical next step was daunting, but it also gave me focus and hope." Unfortunately, laparoscopy isn't cheap—the price runs a few hundred to a few thousand dollars. However, sometimes it is at least partially covered by insurance. (For more information on covering the costs of your infertility, see Chapter 5.)

Hysteroscopy

Like laparoscopy, this procedure requires anesthesia and relies on a lighted telescopelike instrument to guide the way. Only this time around, doctors use it to explore the *inside* of your uterus in search of fibroids, cysts, scar tissues, or structural defects that might be interfering with implantation. While you sleep, the hysteroscope is inserted vaginally—with the aid of a speculum—into your uterus. A hysteroscopy is pretty similar to laparoscopy, except that it usually takes a bit less time since there isn't quite as much terrain to check out.

Getting Your Partner to Go to the Doctor

Now, let's talk about your partner. As mentioned in the first chapter, "male factor" is responsible for roughly 40 percent of all fertility problems. Since the dawn of time, however, the female of the species has usually been the scapegoat for a couple's failure to conceive. Even the father of our country, George Washington, fell into this thinking trap. Though Martha successfully bore children in a previous marriage, she just couldn't get pregnant with George. And, as was the custom of the day, he placed the onus squarely on her. Back then it was believed that a man was only infertile if he was impotent. And George wasn't impotent. Thus, it *had* to be Martha. Today, we know that plenty of men who appear to be fertile are not. We also know that smallpox—which George suffered from as a youth—frequently renders its victims sterile. Alas, there were no fertility doctors around in those days to set the record straight.

But men aren't the only ones in the habit of pointing the finger at women when it comes to fertility woes. We do it to ourselves. Take Trina. This 35-year-old retail manager recalls: "My husband and I tried for two solid years to get pregnant. Because I was six years older than he was, naturally, I assumed it was me. But I went and had every test under the sun and they all came out fine. Then we decided to get Kevin tested, just in case. I still remember my doctor calling with the results, 'Your husband's sperm count is 100,000,' she said. 'Sounds great,' I thought. Then she dropped the bomb—a normal male sperm count is about 100 times that amount. My jaw hit the floor!"

Trina's story illustrates how imperative it is for your significant other to get a complete fertility work-up, too. And for the sake of efficiency, it makes sense for you both to get tested at the same time—even if you strongly suspect that you have a problem. Remember, nearly 20 percent of couples who can't conceive have issues related to both of them. Just as it takes two to tango, it takes two fertile people to have a baby. To make a reasoned decision, or to move forward with IVF, you need all the information you can get.

Where should your partner start? With a good *urologist*—a physician who specializes in disorders of the male reproductive and urinary tract. Ask your general practitioner, gynecologist, or fertility specialist to provide a thoughtful referral. And if your partner is resistant to making an appointment, be patient and convince him of the necessity. Serena, a 26-year-old grad student, recalls the battle with her spouse: "Miguel had a pretty traditional upbringing. I guess you could call him a macho man. It was like a dishonor to seek help. 'If it's meant to be, it will be. I love you with or without kids,' he would say. While that was a lovely sentiment, I really wanted a baby and suspected he did, too. It took six months of coaxing—and I had to set the whole thing up—but he did finally go. And yes, we discovered a problem."

Most men will willingly go to the doctor. But a few will drag their feet, either because they're afraid or ashamed or in denial. In other words, they're human. Accept this reality and work with it. Remember your end game—getting him to go to the doctor so you can find out what's keeping you from getting pregnant. Do what you can to make it happen: Assuage his fears, share facts about male infertility, ply him with a wonderful feast. Men don't hear the ticking of the biological clock as intensely as we do. Give him some time to process his feelings. That being said, don't let the waiting period drag on for too long. You'll need to work as a team to assemble the big picture as well as to navigate the road ahead. (For more strategies on dealing with the emotional aspects of your husband's infertility, see Chapter 4.)

The Basic Fertility Work-up for Your Partner

Like it or not, visits to the doctor sometimes involve some serious waiting. Encourage your partner to make an appointment on a low-impact day. Friday afternoons, when there is little action back at the office, tend to work well. Remind him to take his time to fill out the intake form accurately, be brutally honest, and maintain his sense of humor—the latter may get him through some of the more embarrassing questions.

❧ **Health Problems and Surgeries:** Past and present medical conditions, including mumps after puberty, hernia repairs, even groin injuries, can severely impact fertility. So can sexually transmitted diseases. The doctor should also ask your partner if and when his testicles descended. (Even when surgery is performed during childhood to correct this condition, a man's sperm count is often significantly reduced.) And what about recent fevers? An elevated temperature can lead to low-grade sperm even two months after the fact!

❧ **Medications:** Is your partner taking something that might affect his fertility? Medication for peptic ulcers and high blood pressure, as well as certain antibiotics, can take a toll on sperm counts. In addition, some antidepressants can simply make your partner less inclined to have sex, which is sometimes a factor.

❧ **Sexual Patterns:** Coach your partner to take sex-related questions in stride. Embarrassing as it is to discuss, erectile dysfunction, premature ejaculation, even infrequent trysts can lead to failed conception. In fact, about 5 percent of infertile couples have problems related solely to intercourse. Fortunately, most of these are relatively easy to correct.

❧ **Lifestyle Patterns:** Cigarette smoking, excessive drinking, and chronic marijuana or cocaine use all reduce a healthy sperm count. Anabolic steroids often spell trouble, too. These muscle-growing concoctions actually *decrease* testosterone, ironically rendering some of the most "pumped" guys sterile. Hot tubs anyone? The intense heat is murder on sperm. In addition, extreme exercise—such as riding a bike more than 50 miles a week—can be a significant factor.

Typically, an initial interview is followed by a complete exam. Frank, a 39-year-old sales manager, recalls the experience: "Man, I didn't want to go. I did not want to get squeezed or do *anything* in a cup. I stalled for a long time, but it wasn't all that bad." What can your partner expect? A thorough examination of his penis, prostate gland, and, most importantly, his testicles. (Do references to these body parts make you feel twelve all over again? If so, try to get used to them. They're key players in the fertility game and you may well have to discuss them with both your mate and your RE.) Small, very soft, or misshapen and hard testicles often point to problems with sperm production. Enlargement of the transport tubes behind the testicle, too, can mean there's blockage keeping the sperm from traveling out to the penis and getting you pregnant. Additionally, the doctor should check for signs of *varicoceles*—a group of varicose veins in the scrotum. Why is this a problem? The thinking is that these enlarged veins overheat the sperm, significantly reducing both their quality and quantity. Varicoceles are actually the number one cause of male infertility, accounting for nearly 40 percent of all cases. If the urologist suspects that your partner has this condition, ultrasound can confirm it and surgery—while not always successful—is an option.

Fertility Fact: A recent study at the University of New York at Stony Brook has debunked the notion that boxers are any better than briefs when it comes to increasing sperm count.

I'm sure you've heard the expression, "You can't judge a book by its cover." Well the same holds for a man and his sperm count. A guy can play football, drink beer, love "The Three Stooges," have an incredible sexual appetite, even ejaculate a large quantity of semen, and still have a very low sperm count. In fact, it happens all the time. That's why a thorough semen analysis is the cornerstone of the male fertility work-up. (For a list of other leading tests, see page 44.) As we all know, a semen analysis usually requires a man to masturbate in the not-so-stimulating environs of a lab or doctor's office. Says Jonathan, a 29-year-old financial analyst, "They leave you in this room with a stack of *Playboys* and are like, Go for it! Talk about pressure. At first I had terrible stage fright. But then my sense of humor kicked in—after all this was pretty ridiculous—and I was able to relax and do the job."

Fertility Fact: Sperm accounts for a mere 1 to 2 percent of semen's total volume.

Certainly, it can be a challenge to get in the mood in a bland room featuring a fuzzy Monet print and indoor-outdoor carpeting. Advise your partner to clear his schedule so he doesn't feel pressured by the clock. Tensing up will only make things worse. Also make sure he follows his doctor's instructions to the letter. Most prefer that men abstain from sex for two to four days (but not more!), report recent illnesses (fevers can lower sperm production), capture all their ejaculate (volume is also being evaluated), and, of course, wash their hands thoroughly (bacteria can destroy a sample). What can you do to help? Prepare a few frisky lines and invite him to call you on his cell phone if he is having trouble "rising to the occasion."

Semen Analysis 101

A vial of semen speaks volumes. Here's what doctors are looking at:

✎ **Volume:** Two to 5 milliliters is considered normal. A smaller quantity could point to a production problem or a blocked transport tube.

✎ **Sperm Count:** Forty to 300 million sperm per milliliter is in the normal range; 80 million is average, 20 million is low, and 10 million is very low. That being said, it is still possible to get pregnant with a low or very low sperm count—especially if the sperm's motility and morphology are good. (See below.)

✎ **Motility:** How strong and fast are his swimmers? Lab technicians use high-powered microscopes to see how many sperm are still moving after three hours. Half should be. Sperm are also required to participate in a miniature marathon, in which their progress is tracked across a straight line. If a sizable number show good forward movement—great!—that usually means an adequate number will be able to reach the fallopian tubes, too.

✨ **Morphology:** All sperm are not created equal! Some are immature. Some have two heads or tails. Actually, most don't make the grade. In fact, only 30 out of 100 individual sperm are required to be healthy for a man's sample to pass the morphology test. What's healthy? Sperm with normal heads, midsections, and tails. Is bigger better? Ironically, large-headed sperm are often unable to penetrate an egg.

✨ **Seminal Fluids:** Semen is analyzed for color—it should be a translucent gray—as well as consistency. If it's too thick, the sperm may have trouble swimming out of it to reach the fallopian tubes. Technicians also count white blood cells; more than a million per milliliter could point to an infection or a sexually transmitted disease. Sometimes semen is also cultured to rule out the presence of chlamydia, gonorrhea, and other bacteria.

✨ **Seminal Fructose:** In cases where semen is completely devoid of sperm, doctors check to see if seminal fructose is present. Its absence could point to blocked or missing transport tubes. The latter is a congenital disorder sometimes associated with cystic fibrosis. Thus, if this problem is uncovered, it's essential for men to undergo further testing to determine if they are carriers for the disease.

A sperm is remarkably teeny. Still, it's no bit player in human conception. Without one, a baby simply can't happen.

What can be gleaned from an in-depth study of your partner's microscopic swimmers? Answer: The likelihood that they'll be able to get you pregnant. Following the evaluation, his sperm will get a great, good, so-so, or failing grade (the last in cases where there is no sperm in the ejaculate at all). While there's no question that a high, healthy sperm count maximizes the chances of achieving a speedy pregnancy, a slightly low sperm count can do the job fine—it just might take a bit longer. Poor sperm counts, too, have certainly resulted in pregnancies. But a lower count means that fewer sperm, if any, will make it all the way to the fallopian tubes for possible fertilization. In other words, the cards are stacked against you.

Fertility Fact: In couples with normal fertility, the woman's egg can only be fertilized 12 to 24 hours after ovulation.

What can be done? As mentioned earlier, low or no sperm counts often point to varicoceles or blocked transport tubes, which can often be corrected with microsurgery. Vasectomies, too, can be reversed. All these procedures, however, have varying degrees of success. If surgery is mentioned as a possible remedy, make sure to get a handle on your *real* odds for achieving a pregnancy as well as any waiting period involved. (It generally takes several months before doctors give you the green light to start trying for a baby again.) But even in cases where surgery is not an option, there is still much cause for hope. If a few healthy sperm exist in your partner's epididymis—the tube that stores maturing sperm—or testicles, doctors can extract them with a fine needle for use during in vitro fertilization. This makes the process a bit trickier, of course, but it's still extremely effective. In fact, thousands of babies have gotten their start via this remarkable shortcut.

A Final Word on Figuring Out What's Wrong

I have to admit that pulling together this list of his and her fertility tests brought me down memory lane. That overwhelming feeling of taking the first steps toward solving the mystery of my inability to conceive came flooding back. *Where was I going? How long would my journey take?* Yes, a solid evaluation calls for patience; it can take weeks or months. But it is absolutely vital to your course of treatment—as well as

More Tests for Him

Here's a rundown on some other tests your doctor may want your partner to take:

Hamster–Sperm Penetration Test: No joke, your partner's sperm are combined with hamster eggs. If 15 percent can penetrate the eggs, that's a good sign they can do the same with yours.

Testicular Biopsy: In this test, the doctor removes a bit of tissue from each testicle, then sends it to a lab to see if there are any healthy sperm within it. If some are present, it's conjectured that a blockage is keeping the sperm from exiting the penis.

Vasography: When a doctor suspects a blocked transport tube, a teeny incision can be made in the patient's scrotum. Next, a contrast dye is injected and X-rays taken to sleuth out the trouble spot. This procedure is usually performed under general anesthesia.

Hormonal Evaluation: Just as the right balance of hormones is essential to women's fertility, the right balance of hormones is essential to men's fertility, too. An elevated level of follicle-stimulating hormone, for example, often indicates a sperm production problem. In addition, doctors often check levels of testosterone, luteinizing hormone, prolactin, estradiol, and thyroid-stimulating hormone.

Transrectal Ultrasound: In this test, an ultrasound probe is placed in the rectum to check for blockages, such as cysts, in the ejaculatory duct and seminal vesicles—the two pouchlike glands that produce semen.

Urinalysis: Occasionally, a man's urine is analyzed to see whether it contains semen. If so, this suggests that he's ejaculating backward into the bladder instead of through the penis. When a man has this condition, sperm can sometimes be harvested from his urine for use with IVF.

Antisperm Antibodies: Specific blood and semen evaluations can be ordered to test for the presence of *antisperm antibodies*—antibodies created by the immune system to ward off illness by killing foreign bodies. Sometimes these antibodies attach themselves to sperm, which they mistakenly view as foreign bodies. As a result, the sperm are unable to properly swim and/or penetrate eggs. This condition is common in men with vasectomy reversals.

Karyotyping: In cases of multiple miscarriage, male partners, too, are sometimes asked to undergo an analysis of their chromosomes to check for abnormalities.

your decision to pursue IVF. Marina, a 32-year-old interior decorator, puts it well: "My husband and I tried to get pregnant for two years. I should have gone to the doctor sooner, but I was afraid of all of the exams and needles. And, yes, walking away with confirmation that there was something wrong with me or Tom. But once I got into the process, it was OK. And when we uncovered the fact that I rarely ovulated, I actually felt relieved. Now, at last, we could try to correct it."

Taking the time to figure out what's wrong takes courage and conviction. It's like turning on a light in a room of darkness. And part of you might not want to see what's lurking there. But without illumination, you have no power to right what's wrong. For that reason, I urge you to stay the course, especially if you are 37 or older. Procrastination and missed appointments can lead to reduced fertility as months or years slip by. So take a deep breath, set the goal of finding out what's wrong, and don't forget to pamper yourself during the process—you deserve it. Adriane, a 29-year-old grant writer and now a mom of two, offers this sage advice: "Getting off of the sofa and going to appointments takes guts. I rewarded myself during 'infertility boot camp' with shopping sprees, massages, even the occasional sweet. After each doctor visit, I went out and bought a Cadbury Bar," she recalls with a laugh. "Thinking about it got me through. Don't underestimate the incentive of a great chocolate!"

Chapter 3

Is IVF the Right Choice for You?

ॐ

Choosing the Best Path

To do IVF or not to do IVF? That is the question. Had in vitro fertilization been around in William Shakespeare's era, perhaps he'd have pondered this all-important topic in one of his many plays. Today, it's certainly a subject of heated discussion for millions of couples, though only a fraction of them end up pursuing it. That's mostly good news— a lot of them don't need IVF. Instead, the majority achieve their goal with a less involved solution such as using a fertility drug like clomiphene citrate to improve egg development or pursuing intra-uterine insemination to boost marginal sperm counts. Other couples decide to undergo corrective microsurgeries, skip straight to adoption, or embrace child-free living.

Heard the expression, "No two snowflakes are exactly alike"? Well, the same can be said of in-vitro candidates. Each has a distinct fertility issue, budget, timetable, support system, and frame of mind—all of which must come into play in order to make a reasoned decision. Emily, a 40-year-old data processor, recalls: "When we chose to take a second mortgage out on our house to pay for in vitro, my sister was stunned. She told me I was making a big mistake. But Lou and I carefully thought it through. Our first cycle didn't work, but we're going to try again soon. Do I regret my decision? Not one bit." Emily's story serves to illustrate that in vitro fertilization is a highly personal choice. Should it be yours? This chapter provides information on the range of treatments available to infertile couples. In addition, it offers a quick self-test plus practical assessment tools to help you decide if IVF is the appropriate solution for you.

Exploring Other Options

Following the basic fertility work-up discussed in the last chapter, the cause of a couple's failure to conceive is discovered about 90 percent of the time. Maybe you've got endometriosis, an estrogen deficiency, a compromised fallopian tube, or issues related to your ovarian reserve. Maybe your partner has a hormonal imbalance, varicoceles, or a blocked transport tube. Could be that you're facing a combination of these factors. Or, perhaps there was no great mystery to begin with. It's not unheard of for women who've had tubal ligations or men who've opted for vasectomies to wake up one morning and suddenly find themselves with a raging case of baby fever. All are common scenarios.

The remaining 10 percent of folks who can't readily conceive are considered to have "unexplained infertility," which simply means their doctors can't put their finger on the source of the problem. Cathy, a 36-year-old studio manager, fell into this category: "Over the course of six months, it seems like my husband and I had every test imaginable. At first, every time we 'passed' I was happy. But then it really started to bug me: Why couldn't they figure out what's wrong? In the end, my RE was not able to pinpoint any major cause. Still, he thought IVF might work and, after two cycles, it did. I have to say, having twins certainly makes the diagnosis of unexplained infertility easier to live with." Although the inability to discover the root of your problem can be frustrating, allow yourself to take comfort in the knowledge that it is still quite possible for you to have a baby, either through IVF or a less extensive treatment.

Beth, a 38-year-old accountant, knew why she wasn't getting pregnant, but struggled to choose the best course of action. "Because I was older and had tons of friends who'd done in vitro, I was pretty sure that it was my destiny. But when my doctor checked me out, she thought that I should try a few cycles of Clomid in combination with intrauterine insemination (IUI). Clomid, to help me ovulate, and IUI, to address my husband's slightly low sperm count. Yes, I was worried about my biological clock ticking away during the process, but I agreed to try it three times before graduating to IVF. I'm glad I did. The treatment worked the third time around!"

Beth's story hammers home a key point. It's important for your peace of mind as well as your pocketbook to consider and rule out other lower-tech, less expensive options before pursuing IVF. Otherwise, you may be subjecting yourself to the emotional, physical, and financial obligations of a process that you don't really need. Fact: The vast majority of infertile couples don't require in vitro. They can address their problem with one of the following less demanding protocols.

Fertility Drugs and Timed Intercourse

Clomiphene citrate—brand names Clomid and Serophene—is possibly the most widely used treatment in the world. Around since the 1960s, this oral medication is often the "first line" of offense for women who don't ovulate on a regular basis, especially those with polycystic ovaries. Here's the drill: First, you take Clomid to boost egg development, then you time sex to coincide with ovulation. Clomid is safe and easy with a caveat: Over time, it can temporarily dry up the cervical mucus needed to transport sperm to the fallopian tubes. Therefore, it should not be done for more than three consecutive cycles without a break. If Clomid isn't working, doctors can turn to a host of other, more sophisticated, superovulatory drugs such as Gonal F or Follistim. These, however, are given by injection and require more careful monitoring. Both approaches have succeeded in getting millions of women pregnant.

Intrauterine Insemination with Partner Sperm

Like clomiphene citrate, intrauterine insemination (IUI) has been a staple on the infertility menu for many years. It's a wise therapy for women with poor cervical mucus and/or men with mild male factor.

How does it work? The doctor injects your partner's semen directly into your uterus just prior to ovulation—a simple act that gives his swimmers a huge head start by bypassing your mucus, which may be too thick or contain antibodies that attack and impede their ability to reach your tubes. In addition, doctors are able to give a leg up to nonstellar sperm by "washing them," selecting the best grade, and increasing their quantity by combining two or more samples. This treatment, however, is not recommended for men with moderate to severe male factor; these candidates are well advised to skip directly to IVF. IUI is often done in tandem with the superovulatory medications mentioned above to maximize success rates.

Intrauterine Insemination with Donor Sperm

There is evidence that early scientists began experimenting with artificial insemination as far back as the fourteenth century. Today, it's a sound solution when a partner's sperm count is low or nonexistent. Or, when a single woman or lesbian couple want to conceive. IUI with donor sperm is like regular IUI, only this time the sperm comes from a third party. These days, sperm banks can be accessed via the Internet, enabling you to choose from thousands of candidates. With a few simple keystrokes, you're able to pull up a donor's complete medical history as well as learn about his ethnic background, features, and personality traits—right down to his favorite color and ice cream flavor. When you find a match, the chosen sperm can be purchased and overnighted anywhere in the United States for use in your own doctor's office. Pretty amazing, huh? IUI with donor sperm is an appealing option for some because it's far less expensive and invasive than IVF. Still, the decision to use donor sperm cannot be taken lightly, especially if you have an infertile partner who's struggling with feelings of failure and deep disappointment. Bottom line: This route should be carefully discussed and "lived with" before you pursue it.

Surgeries for You

For women with endometriosis, fibroids, or blocked tubes, microsurgery often clears the way for a healthy pregnancy. However, the operative word here is "often." Success rates hover around 50 percent and don't necessarily add up to a lifetime cure: tubes sometimes get reblocked, growths sometimes come back. For those who've had their tubes tied then—whoops!—changed their minds, reversal surgery is quite common. That being said, your chances of conceiving vary widely depending on the type of procedure you had. The moral of this story is: If you are considering any type of corrective surgery at all, make sure you get a full assessment of your personal odds for achieving pregnancy *before* you commit the considerable time, energy, and financial resources to pursuing it. IVF might prove the better bet.

Surgeries for Your Partner

Microsurgery is a viable option for infertile men with varicoceles as well as transport-tube blockages that are keeping sperm from making their way up and out of the penis. These surgeries tend to be effective about 50 to 60 percent of the time. Ever snicker at a billboard touting vasectomy reversal? Well, it's a big business. This popular surgery often does the trick, but the amount of time that has elapsed since the vasectomy was performed is key. If it was done more than 12 years ago, your chances of getting pregnant are about half of what they'd be if it was done in the past three years. That's because the more years that pass post-surgery, the higher the likelihood of scarring, blockages, and subpar sperm (due to the development of anti-sperm antibodies). It is also important to understand that all of these processes require after-surgery waiting periods of several months to a year to restore a healthy sperm count. If you're 25, that's probably not a problem, but what if you're approaching 40? For these reasons, the pros and cons of each should be weighed against IVF.

Alternative Therapies and Lifestyle Adjustments

Some folks swear by non-Western fertility treatments such as Chinese herbs or acupuncture. And they get results—a recent study suggested that acupuncture boosts natural pregnancy rates by 25 percent! Lifestyle changes, too, can make a big difference. Being severely over- or underweight can cause female infertility, so a regimen of healthy eating and weight adjustment is a wise move if you want to conceive. Also, physical activity is great, but sometimes less is more. Extreme exercise, such as training for a marathon, can temporarily shut down ovulation. And what about stress? Although stress is not a key roadblock to fertility, it certainly causes people to feel lousy, which can dampen couples' sex lives (and, along with it, their baby-making potential). All of this is to say, if you want to get pregnant and have time on your side, consider these inexpensive remedies before graduating to IVF. At least you'll feel better in the process!

Fertility Fact: The nation's first commercial sperm bank opened for business in 1970 in the state of Minnesota.

Now that I've outlined some alternatives to IVF, how do you decide what to do? "It felt like door number one or door number two," said Ken, a 34-year-old contractor. He and his wife Melissa debated their choices—surgery or IVF—then opted for a varicocele repair. After eight months she was able to achieve a natural pregnancy. "The recovery was kind of rough," Ken admits. "But I'm glad we did it. We have one daughter now and can have more the old-fashioned way." Vanessa, a 37-year-old hair stylist, and her husband Scott were not as fortunate. "He went through the surgery, the pain, the waiting period, but no baby. In fact his sperm production is no better now than it was before. So, after all that, we are back to square one. Now, we're gearing up for IVF."

Standing at that fork in the road with one path leading to IUI or microsurgery and the other to IVF is a difficult place to be. If we only had a crystal ball, we would see which way to go. We would know if it were worth devoting a year to IUI, if the tubal surgery would work, or if in vitro offered the best solution after all. Choosing a treatment plan takes clearheaded thinking, patience, and teamwork. It's not a topic to debate with your spouse on the heels of a disappointing test result. Or when you're volatile or teary or irrational or exceptionally depressed. Do these emotions ring any bells? Unfortunately, they are the many moods of infertility. If you're feeling particularly down in the dumps, take a deep breath and set a time to begin talks with your partner the following day. Chances are you'll feel more yourself.

Fertility Fact: The old adage *Just relax and you'll have a baby* is a myth. Although studies show that stress can sometimes affect your ovulation schedule, it is not a factor that will keep you from having a baby.

Make sure, too, that you gather all the facts about your case. Speak to your doctor and ask for his or her candid opinion. (Skilled and experienced REs have definite ideas!) Factors to consider include your age, odds for succeeding, frame of mind, finances, stomach for surgeries, work schedule, and support system. Also, you'll want to be sure that you and your partner are truly on the same page. To help make that call, sit down together and take the following self-test. It's designed to help determine if IVF is the best course of action for you both.

Is IVF Right for Us? Self-Test

1. *Have you exhausted other options and/or ruled them out in a calm and rational state of mind?*

2. *Do you have a clear understanding of the IVF process?*

3. *Do you have a clear understanding of your chances of success, based on your age and fertility issue(s)?*

4. *Do you and your partner agree that it is the very best option for you both?*

5. Does IVF mesh with your moral and religious beliefs?

6. IVF can take several months of time and focus. Can you make that commitment at this point in your life?

7. IVF can cost tens of thousands of dollars. Do you have a plan in place for paying for it? (Funding fertility is covered in Chapter 5.)

8. IVF requires frequent morning visits to the doctor for monitoring. If you have a hectic schedule, will you be able to make all your appointments?

9. Do you feel emotionally prepared to handle IVF, including facing the medical procedures, shots, mood swings, and uncertain outcome?

10. Do you have a support system in place that can help you through the process?

11. At this point, have you carefully considered and ruled out adoption?

12. At this point, have you carefully considered and ruled out living a full life without children?

13. Nearly 36 percent of all successful IVF cycles result in multiple births. Are you prepared for the real possibility that you could become pregnant with twins, triplets, or even quads? Are you aware of the real risks multiples pose to a pregnancy as well as the health of the babies after birth? Are you comfortable with the idea of selective reduction? (This important topic is explored in Chapter 9.)

14. If your cycle succeeds, you will become a parent. Are you ready to face that huge responsibility?

15. *If your cycle fails, you will have to choose a next step. Do you have a loose plan in place for moving forward? Do you have money set aside for subsequent cycles? Are you willing to consider donor eggs or sperm?*

Assessing the Pros and Cons of IVF

Did you or your partner answer "No" to one or more of the questions on the self-test? If so, then it may not be time to make the move to IVF. Because in vitro is an enormous commitment, it's essential that you're both truly ready to pursue it. How do you know when you're *truly* ready? To help clarify your thinking and give you practice making a thoughtful decision, let's analyze the pros and cons of IVF for two hypothetical couples. Although these are not real people, the variables outlined here are similar to those faced by thousands of others—maybe even you.

Here goes:

> *Sue and Peter, both 27, are teachers at the same school. They live in a rental apartment in Baltimore, Maryland. Except for the strain of infertility, they are very content with their life together. After all, there's much to recommend it, including weekend hikes, dinner parties, and loads of nieces and nephews to spoil. Last year they decided they wanted their own baby and stopped using birth control. When Sue didn't get pregnant, they decided to find out if something was wrong. Peter went to a urologist and checked out fine. Sue, however, was diagnosed with mild endometriosis—the likely source of their infertility. Her doctor was able to remove some of it during a laparoscopy. He thinks this will improve their odds of conceiving naturally, but can't make any guarantees. "There's probably a 50–50 chance of your having a baby after a year," is the quote that sticks in their minds. IVF was also mentioned as an option. The doctor thought they'd*

be great candidates, but only half of the procedure would be covered by their insurance. That means they'd have to borrow about $5,000, but from where? Another problem was the risk of multiples. Sue and Peter both agreed that selective reduction—the process of selecting one of the early fetuses for termination—was not an option. But how could they fit twins or triplets in their snug apartment? Sue could do IVF during their summer break, but they'd have to cancel their long-awaited trip to Costa Rica. What should they do?

The Case for IVF:

- The doctor believes they'd be great candidates for IVF.

- Half of the cost of IVF is covered by insurance.

- Sue gets summers off and could do the treatment outside of work.

- Peter is supportive and would be there every step of the way.

- They feel emotionally prepared to face the challenge.

The Case Against IVF:

- They *do* have a 50–50 chance of conceiving naturally.

- Half of the cost of IVF is *not* covered by insurance. They'd have to borrow the rest, probably from their parents. That could be awkward.

- They realize IVF might result in twins and worry about "double trouble" in their little apartment.

- They were really looking forward to their trip to Costa Rica and would rather not miss it.

- They are young enough to put IVF on hold for several years.

Thinking It Through: True, sex the old-fashioned way might not work for Sue and Peter, but there is a 50 percent chance that it *will*. Those are odds a twenty-something couple can work with. Why? If Sue can't manage to get pregnant naturally in a year or two, there'd still be plenty of time to pursue IVF. Putting the treatment on hold would also enable them to save some money to pay for it and/or put a mortgage down on a house. That's a definite plus because if they're required to default onto in vitro and if it succeeds, there's roughly a 36 percent chance of multiples. One final thought: Missing out on a trip to Costa Rica may not sound like such a big deal, but its cancellation could derail the dream for many years to come. After all, if Sue and Peter succeed in achieving a pregnancy, exotic vacations could soon become a thing of the past.

One Conclusion: Try naturally for two years. In the meantime, start socking away some cash for IVF—in case it's needed—as well as to move to a bigger home.

Now, let's look at another hypothetical couple.

Marissa is 39. She recently wed the man of her dreams, 49-year-old J.T., in a mountaintop ceremony. They reside in Taos, New Mexico, where they run a small photography studio. Because J.T. had a vasectomy seven years ago, they knew it would be impossible to conceive on their own. The father of two grown kids, he figured his baby days were over—that is, until he got divorced and met Marissa. Now, they really, really want a baby, but only one. Marissa worried that she might have fertility problems related to her age, but—good news!—all her tests came back in the normal range. When they asked J.T.'s urologist about a vasectomy reversal, he told them it was an option. The chances of the procedure working were good, but it could take a year before a healthy sperm count is restored. The doctor also mentioned IVF, which might prove a more expedient solution. The problem was there was no clinic nearby. A savvy researcher, Marissa was able to locate a great program in

Chicago, Illinois, where J.T.'s parents live. When they flew there for a consultation, they were impressed. The RE they met with told them IVF—with sperm extraction and intra-cytoplasmic sperm injection (ICSI)—was a good bet, but not a sure thing. Turns out, their insurance doesn't cover IVF at all. That means they'd have to break into their nest egg to cover it. What should they do?

The Case for IVF:

- The doctor believes they are good candidates for IVF.

- Since Marissa is 39 it's wise to try to have a baby right away. The vasectomy reversal would require a yearlong waiting period before they could even start trying.

- Because they run their own business, they could close up shop for a while and fly to Chicago for treatment.

- They have enough money saved for a total of four rounds of IVF.

- They are both committed to parenthood and ready to face the challenge of IVF.

The Case Against IVF:

- There are no guarantees that IVF will work for them.

- A vasectomy reversal would be less expensive than even a single round of IVF.

- A vasectomy reversal would enable them to have more kids down the road, provided it worked.

- An IVF pregnancy might result in twins or triplets—a somewhat intimidating prospect.

- They would have to travel to Chicago to pursue IVF treatment, which would require closing their business and living with his parents for several weeks. That could be stressful!

Thinking It Through: Yes, J. T. could have a vasectomy reversal, but what about the several-month waiting period to attempt baby-making? At 39, Marissa's ovarian reserve could become a problem in the near future. On the flip side, if they pursued IVF—and it took four rounds—their hard-earned savings would surely be depleted. But what was the money for anyway? Perhaps the biggest concern a couple like this would face is the risk of multiples. They claim to want only one child. For argument's sake, let's say they talked it through and became comfortable with the idea of selective reduction. (This important topic is covered in Chapter 9.) Dealing with issues such as closing a business, traveling, and, of course, moving in with one's parents during treatment can certainly be taxing. But challenges faced together are often overcome and sometimes have the fringe benefit of making a relationship even stronger.

One Conclusion: Go for it! Skip right to IVF with a rough game plan of pursuing four cycles. If it doesn't work, go back to the drawing board and seriously consider adoption.

A Final Word on Determining Your Game Plan

Would you have drawn the same conclusions as these fictional couples? Blink, and you might. Blink again, and you might not. The decision to pursue IVF is a personal one, often subject to great vacillation. The important thing is that you carefully think it through with the active participation of your partner. Establish some ground rules for making up your minds. Don't try to do it in one sitting, for example. Or when you've had too many cocktails. Or if you're under the influence of extreme emotions. Also, set a time limit for talking about it each day, say a half hour. Too much chat when you're tired can lead to frazzled nerves and fights. Share your feelings freely and encourage your mate to do the same—on a topic of this import, neither of you should feel censored. Your final decision might even surprise you, as was the case with Tess and Jeremy.

"We tried IUI for several months," recounts Tess, a 33-year-old social worker. "When it didn't work, our doctor suggested IVF. At first, we were like, of course we'll do it. But, as we mulled it over, an odd thing happened—both Jeremy and I discovered an urge to help children *already* in the world. The more we thought about it, the more adoption seemed the right choice for us." The epilogue of their story is that they are now the proud parents of a baby girl, adopted in China.

IVF is not for everyone. It's expensive, time-consuming, emotionally draining, and, sadly, sometimes ends in failure. On the other hand, it's nothing short of miraculous for the thousands of people who do it and bring home babies. Is it for you? As mentioned, be sure to carefully weigh the pros and cons aloud with your partner. And read on. Hopefully, this book will provide an in-depth understanding of the process to help you make a secure decision.

Chapter 4

Seeking Emotional Support

ॐ

Are These Feelings Familiar?

They say that men think about sex every seven seconds. Well, I can attest that many women struggling with infertility think about babies with the same frequency and fervor. Take me. I was fine through my mid-thirties, pleasantly preoccupied with a to-do list of scaling the corporate ladder, learning to bake, and jogging along the river. I loved my life. Then I decided to get pregnant. When I couldn't, it was as if some switch got toggled in my brain: Suddenly, all I could think about were babies and the fact that, for now, I couldn't have one. It was pretty depressing. It seemed like every friend was expecting or bouncing a newborn on her knee. I'd go to the mall—babies! I'd go to the museum—babies! I'd go to the park—babies! So, I'd turn on the TV to get some relief, but guess what? On every sitcom and in every commercial, from fabric softener to SUVs—more babies! Babies were taking over the planet! At least that's how it felt at the time.

Sound familiar? The need to procreate is unquestionably primal. It is a desire that consumes us with a ferocity we may never before have experienced. And for many, it's the first time we've ever come face to face with a bona fide life crisis. Puberty, fights with friends, relationship woes, work strife—these are all a cakewalk in comparison. In fact, a recent study found that the levels of depression suffered by infertile couples are tantamount to those of people grappling with life-threatening illnesses such as cancer. Why? Because infertility, like a serious illness, forces us into an uncomfortable limbo-land. Sure, there are positive steps we can take to try to fix things, but these take time. As a result, our lives feel freeze-framed. And we feel powerless.

Sandra, a 32-year-old caterer, recounts: "I was the queen of making order out of chaos. Lobster tortellini for 50? No problem. So, when I couldn't conceive, it really drove me to distraction." Relinquishing our ability to fix things on our own is hard. We're forced to be patient—even when we want resolution now. We're forced to be proactive—even when we're feeling low. "The inability to conceive affects all aspects of a person's life," stresses Carole Lieber Wilkins, a Los Angeles therapist who specializes in fertility issues. Sound like an overstatement? Take a look at how infertility stretches its tentacles into every facet of our being:

☙ **Sense of Self:** If we can't have a baby, who are we? Infertility often triggers feelings of low self-esteem. Women beat themselves up with questions such as "What's wrong with my body?" or "Why didn't I try to have a kid when I was 21?" Men may begin to see themselves as less virile because their sperm can't do its essential job.

☙ **Relationships:** Struggling to conceive puts undo stress on a marriage or partnership. The two of you may have diametrically opposed ideas on the best way to solve your problem. That can lead to fighting. Or, you may start to blame each other. Connections to parents, siblings, and friends—the very people you need to lean on the most—can suffer too, buckling under the strain of perceived insensitivity and/or jealousy.

☙ **Sexuality:** For some, the onset of infertility turns sex into a mid-cycle chore—suddenly intercourse is on par with brushing one's teeth. For others, the reality that a lovemaking session cannot result in a pregnancy simply dampens their enthusiasm for the event. Either way, two life-sustaining aspects of sex—intimacy and bodily pleasure—often fall by the wayside.

☙ **Employment:** Managing a career and fertility treatments is quite a balancing act. What do you say, for example, when your boss skeptically ask why you need to take *more* time off for *another* doctor's appointment? In addition, sadness can spill over into the office, making it hard for you to concentrate and do quality work.

৵ **Finances:** IVF costs anywhere from $1,000 to $50,000, depending on your insurance coverage and the number of cycles you'll need. If you're lucky enough to have some money tucked away for a rainy day—when infertility strikes, believe me, it's raining. The rest will have some serious number-crunching and decision-making to do.

৵ **Future:** Infertility has a funny way of putting your life on hold. You can't switch jobs because it will affect your insurance coverage. You can't commit to an evening cooking class because you're saving for treatments. You can't take a much-needed vacation because it conflicts with your IVF start date. Planning for the future—or even tomorrow—begins to feel like an impossibility.

৵ **Sense of Fairness:** Most of us are brought up to believe that life is fair. After all, America is a democracy. Therefore, it's very hard to come to terms with the injustice of being denied what feels like a fundamental human right—having a child.

৵ **Sense of Fun:** Suddenly, the simple joy of a spring day eludes us. We don't feel spontaneous or light on our feet. There is so much heaviness, it's hard to summon strength for the little things that used to bring us so much pleasure.

No doubt everyone's experience with infertility is different. For some, it moves in like the houseguest from hell—following them from room to room, taking over their lives. Others seem to weather the storm with greater ease. Take Ava, a 29-year-old med student: "We had a male factor, but we stayed upbeat and were confident that IVF would work," she practically chirped. "After two cycles it did."

Yes, a lucky few breeze through the process with minimal discomfort. (I hope you are one of them.) However, dealing with infertility is a challenging prospect for everyone to a greater or lesser degree.

But you *do* retain some control. There are steps you can take to gar-
ner loving support from your family and friends. There are steps you
can take to form a united front with your partner. There are even
steps you can take to beat those raging but-I-want-a-baby-now blues.
(I remember them well.) Rest assured, there is much, much reason
to be hopeful, even if you can't summon that particular feeling right
now. This chapter is here to help you maintain a crucial sense of
equilibrium as you move toward your goal of bringing home a baby.

Strategies for Keeping Your Emotions in Check

Before we move on to relationship issues, it makes sense to devote a
little more time to those industrial-strength emotions that plague so
many of us. When infertility hits, our moods seem to come in more
colors than a 64-count box of Crayola Crayons. First there are the
blues: feelings of sadness, desperation, isolation, and bone-tired
weariness from months of disappointment. Then there are the
greens: unbridled jealousy of sisters and cousins and colleagues with
kids—even complete strangers that parade their perfect babies down
the street in fancy carriages just to spite us (or so it seems). Then,
there are the reds: pure, fire-stoked rage at your insurance carrier
for not covering treatments, at your friends for not understanding
the depths of your despair, at your body for not delivering on its
promise. Finally, there are the yellows: those occasional bursts of
hope that nurture our spirits and keep us optimistic. Those sunny
jolts that remind us that, with treatment, our dreams of babies are
real possibilities.

Infertility has a funny way of getting us in touch with feelings we
didn't even know we had. While that may be good for actresses who
have to emote on cue, a tumultuous mind-set can sap our strength
and interfere with our ability to maintain our lives and pursue our
treatment plans. So how do you take the reins and keep your emotions from controlling you? Ironically, perhaps the best tip I can give
you is to try *not* to control them at all. If you don't believe me, take

this quick test. Ready? *Don't* picture a bowl of apples, grapes, and bananas on a wooden table. OK, is the image firmly emblazoned in your mind's eye? I thought so. The same holds true for emotions. The more we command ourselves not to experience them, the more we will. Denying our feelings, beating them down, or shaming ourselves because we have them will only serve to make them worse.

Dylana, a 37-year-old office manager—and now a mom—recalls: "During my two years of IVF treatments, I swear, there were a million and one baby showers. Every cousin, neighbor, and coworker was expecting. The hardest was my best friend's pregnancy. Yes, I was happy for her, but I was very jealous, too. I hid it well or so I thought. That is, until her shower rolled around. Things went fine until someone gave her a little cradle with a baby blue gingham lining. It was something about that fabric. I lost it and ran from the room crying. I felt so humiliated." Ahhhh, those blissful baby showers—the recurrent nightmare of most infertile women. Not only are they a reminder of what we don't have (a baby), they can also be a source of great self-recrimination when envy rears its ugly head.

What should you do? There are a variety of strategies, but here's one that I found worked for me: I'd shake hands with that emotion and sit myself down for a little chat. *Yes, I'd say, you're feeling ferociously jealous that it's not you in the chair being celebrated today. After all you're the one who's fighting to have a kid. All she had to do was have sex! But you know your infertility is not her fault and her having a baby doesn't preclude your having one, too. She's a great person and she deserves it.* Did that impromptu tête-à-tête make my mood bright as a spring day? Not really. But it did keep my emotions from bubbling over into the danger zone. Making a conscious effort to intellectualize what you are going through enables you to be your own therapist. It acknowledges your deep sadness and helps steer your behavior in the right direction. I know these internal dialogues sound a bit corny, but they did get me through some tough times.

They came in particularly handy on those mornings I didn't believe I had the strength to even get out of bed. My wiser self would say, *You're feeling really low. I know you just want to pull the covers up over your eyes and stay here forever. But you really will feel better if you get up and shower and go meet your friends for brunch.* Sometimes, a conversation like that would be enough to get me going, albeit sluggishly at first. And the truth was, I *did* feel better. The fresh air soothed me. The support of my friends nurtured me. And I even laughed at a joke or two, which made me part of the land of the living again. My point: As hard as it is, try to motivate your body to do the things it enjoys and your mind may follow its lead.

Fertility Fact: Research shows that the levels of depression faced by infertile people are as high as those dealing with life-threatening illnesses.

But also cut yourself some slack, especially when it comes to baby showers and baby-centric gatherings. Women report that the winter holidays are especially rough. "Over the years, I'd lost sight of the fact that Christmas is *about* the birth of a baby," reports Laura, a 29-year-old mortgage broker currently saving toward IVF. "Images of mother and child are everywhere! Then, there's the traditional dinner at my mom's house. In come all my nieces decked out in velvet dresses and looking too cute for words. Don't get me wrong, I really love them. But each was a reminder of what I didn't have."

Therapist Carole Lieber Wilkins advocates giving yourself permission to opt out of such events if they are just too painful. After all, you won't be much of a party guest if you're living in fear of a meltdown. Check in with yourself on all upcoming occasions to figure out if you should attend. Are you going to be OK at the christening of your brother's son? How about that Fourth-of-July picnic with all of those toddlers running around? Addressing your infertility is a challenging process—you don't need to add to the burden by forcing yourself to become an emotional superhero. If possible, call up your loved one or friend and let him or her know that you'd really like to be there, but it's just too hard right now. Chances are they'll understand. Chances are they'll appreciate your honesty. For more tips on enlisting the support of friends and family read on.

Getting Help from Family and Friends

Although it's perfectly clear to you that you're suffering from a raging case of the I-wanna-baby blues, it's probably perfectly *unclear* to the rest of the world. I remember how I felt at the beginning of my fertility treatments: ready, willing, and able to burst into tears at the mere mention of a coworker's pregnancy. Or when my sister hugged her daughter. Or when couples with kids made those cute, self-deprecating remarks about family life. I'll never forget the beauty uttered by my friend Sheila over the phone one day, "You don't know how lucky you are to be able to see all the movies and Broadway shows you want," she said with a laugh (her little boy whimpering in the background). "With the baby, Craig and I *never* get to go out anymore. When you have a child your life just does a complete 180." Amazing how a seemingly innocuous remark can set off a private firestorm. What she was trying to communicate was, "My life has changed. I wish I could get out more." What I heard was "We are so lucky to have a kid. You don't have one. You're not in the club. Nah, nah!" I hung up the phone and swallowed my tears. But they resurfaced that evening in bed as I fumed to my husband about her flagrant insensitivity. Then he pointed out that Sheila had no clue we were experiencing fertility problems. How could I expect her to be sensitive to our situation if she didn't even know what our situation was? He was right. I resolved to call her the next day and give her the heads-up.

And I did. Breaking the news was tricky. How do you segue from "Nice weather we're having" to "I'm in the midst of a personal crisis"? Somehow, though, I managed to get the words out. No surprise, she was utterly stunned and truly sorry about her comments. She was also sorry that she had not been more supportive. But how could she have been? She wasn't psychic. Sometimes our own pain is so visceral, we actually trick ourselves into thinking others can feel it, too. They usually can't. And even if they *do* sense something is wrong, more likely than not they'll choose to say nothing out of respect for our privacy. As Sheila and I talked on, I began to feel better. She pledged to help me out during my treatments, even if it was just to get together for low-fat, decaffeinated lattes so I could vent. It felt good that she cared.

After my minidrama with Sheila, my husband and I decided to re-think our strategy of whom to tell. A few months before, we'd made a pact to share our problem with no one except our parents. As supportive as they were, I was beginning to realize their love and attention was not enough to sustain me. Plus, our little secret left me feeling isolated and closeted. Why should I feel ashamed that my body wasn't doing what I wanted it to? At the same time, I didn't relish having to provide monthly status reports to everyone from my second-cousin-once-removed to the guy behind the counter at the dry cleaners. And I didn't want the world feeling sorry for me. Nevertheless, I *did* want to share the general facts of my situation with a few more carefully selected friends and family members. I wanted them to understand what I was going through. And the truth was, I craved their support.

Tips on Who to Tell

It's a big decision to decide who to share your struggle with. Some couples are comfortable opening up to just about everyone, while others prefer to keep their personal life under lock and key. In the end, we decided that something in between felt just right for us. So who made our to-tell list? First and foremost, our siblings. They suspected something was up, but were afraid to ask. This infused our get-togethers with a screaming silence. We'd go out for pizza and it was like a pink elephant was seated at the head of the table, but nobody said a word. Telling them made the elephant disappear. Next, I chose two old friends (in addition to Sheila) whom I knew to be upbeat and sensitive. I also chose a new friend—a woman I'd met at the gym who was very open about her own experience with IVF. After two years of trying, it worked and she gave birth to twins. I figured she'd be a great mentor. My husband, meanwhile, selected a buddy who'd helped him through some tough times in the past. Then came the wild card—an elderly neighbor who had a knack for saying exactly the right thing at the right time. She turned out to be a godsend. Just hearing her warm voice instantly calmed us. Finally, we each confided in a trusted colleague at work. We figured we might need allies to occasionally help us navigate office politics and just be there when we needed them.

No, we didn't call everybody up that night and fill them in on every twist and turn of our struggle. That wouldn't have been constructive or realistic. But over the course of a few weeks, we took a couple minutes to give each of them a heads-up, and in so doing, the permission to be there for us. Along the way, we also shared our story with a few more people when it just seemed right. In all cases, I was amazed at how responsive people were. *Everyone* wanted to know how they could help.

For many, this was the first time they'd ever been called upon to be supportive to someone in the throes of infertility so they didn't have any road map to follow. I didn't have a road map either, but I reflected on what I was feeling and spoke from the heart. I told them I didn't want them to walk on eggshells around me, but I'd appreciate—even welcome—occasional queries about how it was going.

Fertility Fact: A recent poll found that nearly 70 percent of Americans are in favor of in vitro fertilization.

That would let me know they cared. I wanted them to understand I might be a little down on occasion and that was OK. Putting on a counterfeit smile 24/7 can get pretty taxing. But most importantly, I asked them to treat me, well, like *me*. Yes, my infertility was a huge issue in my life at the moment, but it wasn't the sum of my parts. I still liked reading biographies. I still liked joking around. I still liked spending Saturday afternoon wandering the stalls of the local flea market. Continuing on with my life seemed the right thing to do and helped remind me that I already had much to be thankful for.

Letting a few key people in on our secret proved to be a wise decision for us. Should you do the same? That's a question that only you can answer. Everyone is unique and has a distinct style of navigating their interpersonal world. Listen to your instincts, but also acknowledge the fact that no one can help you when they're in the dark. Who *should* you tell? Anyone who you gauge will offer support, including friends, family, neighbors, clergy members, coworkers, even bosses (provided you have the right rapport with them).

Who *shouldn't* you tell? Anyone who you gauge *won't* offer support. That's a mistake that Linda, a 34-year-old receptionist, won't make again: "At a family dinner I told my aunt that we were planning to undergo IVF. Bad idea! We were really close, but she's deeply religious and opposed to any kind of medical intervention when it comes to infertility. After that, she kept trying to convince me that my decision was wrong and kept saying it should be in God's hands."

A recent study shows that 70 percent of Americans are in favor of IVF. That's good news, but what about the other 30 percent? If you suspect a friend or family member will be opposed to your treatment plan, why open up that can of worms by telling them in the first place? Who else should you cross off your to-tell list?

- People who might be uncomfortable with these intimate details of your life and simply won't know what to say.

- People who love to gossip. That is, unless you want the whole world to know your business.

- People with a seeming sixth sense for making insensitive remarks. You know the ones, "Wow. It only took me a month to get pregnant" or "You're overreacting. Just relax and let it happen naturally."

If I had a nickel for every time I heard that last one! Which brings me to a final point. What should you do when a friend or family member says something that sticks in your craw to the point of making your blood boil and/or your eyes well up with tears? As I mentioned before, sometimes loved ones hurt us unwittingly. The topic of infertility has been tiptoed around for so long, a lot of well-intentioned folks fumble for the right words, then inevitably come up with the wrong ones.

Other times, though rarely, people are just plain mean. Either way, when someone says something inappropriate, you have two options— get over it or educate them. If you feel there is no way to get through to them, it's probably best to simply walk away. And accept that they just don't get it. If, however, you sense an opportunity to help them reflect on their statements, choose education. First, count to five so you can get a grip. Then calmly tell them—a minute or a few days later—why you found their remark so hurtful. Chances are they will welcome your honesty and the opportunity to revise their behavior down the road. Chances are you'll feel better, too. Dealing head-on with troubling comments helps them to dissipate so you can focus on the more important goal of achieving a pregnancy.

You and Your Partner, a United Front

Now, on to your greatest ally during infertility treatments—even if it may not always feel that way—your significant other. I'm not big on pop-psychology paradigms, but when it comes to infertility it *can* seem like men are from Mars, women are from Venus. Although there are many exceptions to the rule, women tend to be utterly consumed with the problem. We eat, sleep, and breathe baby-making. It's as if an infertility fairy is sitting on our shoulder whispering in our ear at every moment. Therapist Carole Lieber Wilkins says, "A woman who can't conceive tends to be very focused on the goal. It can feel like war. It can feel like life or death." Meanwhile, her partner may appear to be going about his day-to-day living, business as usual. She sees him head out the door with his buddies to play golf. She catches him humming a tune and wonders how he can be upbeat in the midst of a life crisis. Sure, your partner *says* he wants a baby, but the quest doesn't seem to be consuming him as it does you.

That's what Cara thought. This 40-year-old graphic designer reports: "After two years of struggling to get pregnant, our doctor called us in to tell us he'd discovered a major problem with my husband's sperm. IVF would be our only option. I remember the ride back from his office. I was so miserable, so stressed out. Then I looked over at my husband—driving along in stony silence, his face an emotionless mask. Finally, I couldn't take it anymore and I screamed, 'You don't even care!' To which he responded, 'I'm devastated.' Lightning flash: I suddenly realized the mask meant that he *was* in pain. After that, whenever I saw it, I knew he needed me."

Don't assume because your partner doesn't fall to the ground kicking and screaming that he doesn't care. The reality is that most men want children just as much as we do. They just don't show it in the same way. Blame it on cultural conditioning. Blame it on the Y chromosome. But recognize that men are far more likely to internalize their grief and shift it into low gear than we are. Although your partner may be the atypical type who sobs when watching *Titanic*, chances are he's less overtly emotional than you are. In fact, it's altogether possible he's attempting to fix your infertility in the same way he'd approach a leaky faucet—calmly, through a series of methodical steps.

While this may seem anathema to a woman on the verge of throwing plates, realize that it's a highly effective coping strategy. He may, for example, express worry about financing IVF—crunching and re-crunching the numbers to see if you can afford it. While your strategy—also valid—might be to beg, borrow, or steal to secure funding. Know that his concerns are actually legitimate. If possible, harness his cool-headedness and use it to your advantage. How? Let him do some of the legwork to help solve your problem by researching local IVF practices online or calling your insurance provider to find out what is and isn't covered. Don't try to make him into someone he's not. But do involve him in the process in ways that play to his strengths. You really need to help each other now.

Getting on the Same Page

OK, you might be saying to yourself, respecting each other's perspective is all well and good, but what do you do when you're not even close to seeing eye-to-eye? Consider Holly's situation. This 34-year-old English teacher shares, "When I heard we couldn't have kids naturally, I was *so* ready to do IVF. But my husband didn't feel the same. He hates invasive technology and didn't like the odds. He felt *very* strongly that we could have a full life without kids. We were not only on different pages—we were in completely different books."

Marie's disagreement with her husband was different in nature, but nonetheless challenging. This 44-year-old school administrator recalls: "After a few failed cycles of IVF, my doctor informed me that, because of my age, my chances of conceiving were very slim unless I used an egg donor. That statement felt like a kick in the stomach. I wasn't ready to hear 'donor egg.' When I discussed it with my husband, he thought it was a good option—which made me even madder. How could he be so quick to jump on the bandwagon? A donor egg was a big step. I know my husband meant well, but his enthusiasm hurt. It felt disloyal."

Sometimes it happens that a couple has diametrically opposed opinions on how (or even whether) to proceed with IVF. As hard as it seems, remind yourself that there is no absolute truth here. Your partner's perspective is legitimate and he has a burning need to be heard—just as you do. Try to squint through the haze of your fervor to see his viewpoint. As previously discussed, this can often be achieved by setting aside some time to present both of your opinions in a calm, rational discussion. Don't try to talk when you're so angry you can't see straight. Also, don't overdo the conversation at any one sitting. Stick to the rule of a half an hour a day several times a week. And if the negotiations get overheated, reach for these invaluable tools: reason, patience, compromise, love.

Chances are that continued conversation—free of drama and cutting remarks—will lead to a sensible plan that works for both of you. And if talks break down completely, seriously consider couples counseling. Although this may seem a drastic step, know that infertility can rip at the fabric of the strongest marriage. Address your problem before it's too late with a good therapist who has experience treating infertility issues. If all goes well, he or she will prove to be a great sounding board and advocate for both of you. (For more about selecting a therapist, see page 77.)

Salvaging Your Sex Life

When infertility strikes, lovemaking can suddenly feel about as intimate as rubbing two sticks together. Listen to Carmen, a 32-year-old
customs broker: "My husband and I always had a great sex life. That
is, until I started trying to get pregnant. Then it was bye-bye spon-
taneity and hello timed intercourse. We were doing it so often, I literally *did* begin to have headaches." Attempted baby-making often
starts out with a bottle of wine and sweet talk of baby booties whis-
pered into a lover's ear. But as the weeks unfurl and the pressure
mounts, it can devolve into an act as mechanical as doing the dishes.
Forget abandon. Forget orgasms. There's nothing like a diagnosis of
infertility to turn the joy of sex into the misery of failed conception.
It's ironic, but just when you most need a deep physical connection
to your partner, your love life may start to go to hell.

"Couples have trouble sorting sex into the two categories of procreation and recreation," points out therapist Carole Lieber Wilkins.
Lines get blurred. Agendas get confused. The female partner may be
angry that her husband still wants sex, despite their crisis; the male
partner may be mad that she only wants to do it to make a baby. (And
believe it or not, he can even start to feel pretty objectified.) This
causes hurt feelings and resentment on both sides.

What can you do about it? Set aside the time to have sex just for the
sake of having sex. That means no ovulation ambush for your mate; no
baby-making agenda for you. That may also mean getting away for a romantic weekend stockpiled with your favorite activities such as sunning
and hiking and eating fine food. In some cases these sensory touchstones can awaken your seemingly dormant sexuality by reminding you
of the good things life has to offer—including foreplay, orgasms, and
languid embraces. Some people unwittingly punish themselves for
their inability to conceive by denying themselves access to pleasure.
Don't fall into this trap. Give yourself the stuff you love, whether it's
tickets to a Bruce Springsteen concert or a lazy Sunday morning in bed
with your partner. You deserve them now more than ever.

Also, share you feelings with your partner. No one wants to talk
about his or her sex life ad nauseam, but acknowledging the exis-

tence of a temporary problem sometimes serves to take the edge off. Finally, as odd as it sounds, try to maintain your sense of humor. "Our sex life took a nose dive when I got really focused on having a baby," comments Arianna, a 29-year-old advertising copywriter. "My husband would say, 'Sex again? I feel like a piece of meat.' That made us both laugh. His humor was always a turn-on for me, so his jokes relaxed me and improved our sex life." The truth is intercourse may be a self-conscious act for a while. It may feel staged. It may even carry a tinge of sadness—especially for those who can't rely on its magic alone to deliver a baby. Soothe yourself with the knowledge that your fertility issue will resolve itself in time. And when it does your sex life should return to its normal course.

Avoiding the Blame Game

Remember "for better or worse"—that golden sound bite from your wedding ceremony? Remember believing it with all your might? Well, sometimes the onset of infertility causes us to lose sight of that little contract. Blinded by frustration and rage, we can manage to say some pretty destructive things. Carrie, a 41-year-old attorney, recounted to me one of her low points: "My husband and I were having a fight, basically because we were pissed off that we couldn't have a kid. And I blurted out something like, 'If only we had tried five years ago when I first suggested it, but NO you had to wait till the timing was just right. So much for your perfect timing!' His face fell. I couldn't believe I'd said something so hurtful, especially since we'd both arrived at that decision together."

A friend of mine who's a kindergarten teacher decompresses conflict by reminding kids to count to five before they lash out at classmates. Often, that five-second waiting period is enough for children to decide *not* to make the statement they had planned. It sounds like a simplistic solution, I know, but sometimes it works—even with adults. If you feel like you're boiling over and that zinger is on the tip of your tongue, count to five and try to swallow it. Then, reconsider. For example, instead of saying, "If only *you* hadn't insisted on taking a new job with *lousy* insurance, we would have our IVF treatments completely paid for!"—you might substitute "Infertility *sucks!*" After all, that's probably what you're feeling. Then blow off steam with a run in the park or fury-fueled scrubbing of the bathtub. (It probably needed it anyway.) But what about those statements that really, really must come out? Consider venting to an impartial girlfriend, a therapist, or, better yet, a journal. "My journal was my lifesaver," reports Debbie, a 43-year-old bookseller. "It gave me a safe place to put all of my thoughts." Sometimes the very act of setting free those taboo feelings is enough to defuse them. Then you can analyze them for what they really are—usually free-floating rage at the unfairness of your predicament.

Fertility Fact: A Swedish research report showed that the marriages of couples who underwent IVF were as strong or stronger than those of couples with no fertility problems.

Now, a word on another staple of infertility—self-blame. No doubt you've experienced this firsthand. I'd wager that your partner has, too. Many men, especially with male infertility issues, are plagued with tremendous guilt. Mark, a 44-year-old civil engineer, remembers, "When Jen's arm was black and blue from all the sticks related to our treatment, I felt terrible. It was as if she was paying the price for my low sperm count." No one likes seeing their loved ones in pain. Even if your partner hasn't verbalized feelings of guilt, it doesn't mean he hasn't experienced them. Give him the assurance that you don't blame him by peppering your infertility conversations with phrases like, "We're in this together" or "You've really been there for me." He may need to hear it.

One would be hard-pressed to say there is a silver lining to infertility. In my opinion, it would be nice if everyone could skip to the happily-ever-after of having a healthy baby. However, if you *can* weather the storm together, chances are it will make your relationship stronger, more intimate, and better equipped to handle the other surprises life has in store.

A Word for Single Women Pursuing IVF

Although the majority of people who pursue IVF are couples, a number of single women choose to do it as well. That's not surprising. What is surprising, however, is that just 10 years ago a number of the most prestigious practices in the United States refused to treat them. The thinking was that single women didn't have the essential support system in place to get through the process and/or effectively raise children. Let me climb on my soapbox for one minute and say, Shame! In this day and age, families take many forms. If you are solo and considering IVF, know that thousands of single women have managed the treatments just fine and brought home healthy babies to loving, nurturing homes. Know, too, the tide is turning. Today, nearly 85 percent of the nation's 400 infertility practices accept single women (and those numbers are on the rise). So hang in there, get support, and go for it!

Five Ways to Feel Better As You Await IVF

1. Take a trip

2. Keep a journal

3. Exercise

4. Do yoga

5. Join a support group or try therapy

Thinking About Therapy

You may be planning on plunking down thousands of bucks on IVF. You may be devoting countless hours a week to doctors' visits. So it's easy enough to conclude that therapy is simply not worth the added expense or time commitment. One of the most insidious aspects of infertility is that, because it's so overwhelming, many fail to seek the help they genuinely need. Sure, therapy may drain a few more dollars and eat up another hour of your busy week. But if you really need it—and many IVFers find that they do—it may prove to be an invaluable pressure release.

Take Mollie. This 34-year-old science teacher was resistant to getting help, but her husband changed her mind. "It was New Year's Eve and I'd just gone through an IVF cycle, which failed. At a big family party, I remember my uncle raising his champagne glass at midnight and toasting the four babies born to our extended family that year. I remember him saying, 'Here's to our four hopes for the future.' Everybody cheered, but I felt like I'd been sucker punched. I felt like a nobody because I was childless. I immediately grabbed a champagne bottle and downed about five glasses. The next morning I awoke to a wicked hangover and my husband's voice telling me I needed to get help. I was in no position to disagree." For Janey, a 32-year-old artist, her deep depression crept up on cat feet: "Every week that passed without a pregnancy made me more world-weary. Until, one day, I tried to go out for a run, but didn't have the energy to get around the block. What happened to the health-conscious, fun, spontaneous me, I thought? I have to find a way to feel better."

Infertility is a disease with a host of nasty symptoms, including depression, frustration, isolation, exhaustion, marital discord, low self-esteem, and self-medication to the point of abuse. Sure, you may get away with a mild case and only have to face one of these. Or, you may get clobbered with all of them at the same time. How do you know when it's time to get help? Susan O'Brecht, a New York City therapist who's treated a number of infertile patients, warns people to be on the lookout for these red flags:

• You can't focus at work.

• You're eating too much or too little.

• You're sleeping too much or too little.

• You're feeling helpless or hopeless.

• You're drinking excessively or self-medicating with drugs.

• You're having trouble relating to your spouse, friends, or family.

• You're utterly stuck and can't make a decision regarding treatment.

If any one of these red flags hits home, consider picking up the phone and getting help. Therapy is often at least partially covered by medical insurance—especially when the culprit is infertility—so be sure to check your policy. Make sure as well that you locate a therapist who is sensitive to your needs. When interviewing candidates, Susan O'Brecht advises that you ask if they've treated people whose primary issue was infertility. "It's not essential they have firsthand experience, but it is essential that they have dealt with the specifics of this life crisis," she says. To find a therapist, ask for a referral from your fertility practice (if you have one) or get in touch with Resolve. Resolve, a nonprofit organization dedicated to helping people overcome infertility, maintains a database of experienced counselors across the United States. Contact your local chapter for a list, via their Web site or by calling the national help line. (See the sidebar on page 82 or the *Resources* section at the back of the book for contact information.)

Fertility Fact: Although feelings of deep sadness can strike at any time, people experience the greatest degree of depression in the small hours of the morning. If you've hit rock bottom at 5:30 A.M., know that you may well feel a lot better by noon.

What can you expect to accomplish with therapy? "It wasn't a quick fix," reports Monica, a 37-year-old personal trainer. "I still had to work through a lot of pain. But it did help me focus on my goal. It also gave me a place to vent—a place to explore everything I was feeling without judgment or shame." No, counseling isn't a panacea, but a good therapist should be able to provide you with solid strategies for coping with day-to-day living, ironing out wrinkled relationships, and crafting an action plan. There's just one caveat: Be sure to set some basic objectives for your sessions, including a game plan. Unlike many other life issues, infertile women must contend with their biological clocks. For that reason, it's wise to decide on a reasonable timetable for moving forward with IVF before it's too late.

Connecting with the IVF Community

If you're like I was, you're probably burning to talk to other card-carrying members of the infertility club. As mentioned earlier in this chapter, I made it my mission to strike up a friendship with a nice woman at the gym after she mentioned that her twin girls were courtesy of IVF. The bid for her attention was so calculated that it kind of felt like high school all over again. No matter. She was thrilled to be able to help and had great advice on everything from picking a good practice (she'd been to three) to administering intramuscular injections (she'd given herself dozens). Frankly, I don't know how I would have gotten through the process without her. Plus, she was a living, breathing example that IVF does work.

So how do you go about finding a mentor or sister in the struggle? I don't suggest you approach that stranger who bolted from that baby shower when the booties were displayed. (Maybe it was just bad shrimp.) But I do suggest you seek out women who have been open about their fertility treatments—even if you barely know them. Has a friend of a friend had success with IVF? A cousin? How about a coworker? Ask someone who knows that person well to ask her if it's OK for you to approach her for advice. Chances are she'll respond with an enthusiastic yes. The fact of the matter is that most IVF veterans are more than happy to play senior to your freshman by offering sage advice and tips from the trenches. If possible, arrange to meet them for lunch or make a phone date. You'll be surprised at how shared infertility is an instant icebreaker. And who knows, you may even become lifelong friends.

Another place to turn for information and emotional support are Resolve support groups. These weekly meetings are a great, great forum for infertile women—and men—to meet, open up, and share triumphs and tragedies. Stephanie, a 31-year-old coffee-shop manager, had this to say: "I was truly at my wit's end. My joy was depleted. My marriage was in pretty bad shape. Then, a friend told me about a support group, so I went. It was like Eureka! Here were a dozen women going through the same thing as me. They listened. They understood. And each meeting made me stronger." Resolve has chapters all across the country and holds meetings in dozens of cities and towns. To find out where and when, get in touch with your local chapter.

But if support groups aren't your cup of tea or if you live in a remote location—fear not—you can still connect with the infertility community via your trusty computer. Inside the cyber walls of customized chat rooms, you'll find dozens of women grappling with the inability to conceive—many with profiles very similar to yours. (See *Resources* for some choice Web sites.) Some are looking to impart wisdom; some are looking for a shoulder to lean on. You can even hook up with a buddy who's going through IVF at the same time as you. Here's Yolanda, a 42-year-old homemaker: "I live in rural Nevada, but I connected with a woman who lived in Detroit. We both did in vitro at the same time and compared notes the whole way through. She got pregnant on her first try; I got pregnant on my third. But we still stay in touch. I hope to meet her face-to-face one day, our kids in tow."

There's no question that the Internet is a great source of companionship and information. I'd just like to share a few quick pieces of advice. First, when conducting research, be sure to check the copyright date on material you're devouring. The Internet is an amazing tool, but it is also rife with outdated facts (like the call for boxer shorts). Since IVF is a moving target, even text from the late 1990s is likely to be obsolete. Second, beware of the unscrupulous pitchmen preying on infertile people with promises of amazing miracle cures. If a fertility product sounds too good to be true, chances are it's the modern-day equivalent of snake oil. Third, Web sites and chat rooms are wonderful places to connect with the IVF community. But they can also become a serious addiction. Try to resist the temptation to spend every waking moment online, to the detriment of your job, your relationships, and the quality of your life.

About Resolve (www.resolve.org or 888–623–0744): Founded in 1974, this national nonprofit has helped thousands of people *resolve* their infertility via a dedicated help line, infertility magazine, referrals to reproductive endocrinologists and therapists, and scores of support groups. Resolve is also a powerhouse lobbying group fighting to improve insurance coverage for IVF and other fertility treatments. If you'd like to learn more, visit their Web site. It's loaded with information and resources, plus has a great bulletin board. Membership dues are $55 a year.

A Final Word on Taking Care of Yourself

I hope this chapter has provided some solid strategies to help manage your moods as you navigate your way to and through IVF. Infertility is a tough road. Don't forget to be kind to yourself during the journey. And to get help from friends and family. Work with your partner, not against him. And don't deprive yourself of the things you love, whether they're an expensive haircut or a slice of chocolate-chip cheesecake.

Also, be true to your own personal style. When it comes to IVF, there seem to be two basic personality types. Some women shift into high gear and channel all their nervous energy into researching every corner of infertility science, until they're practically a Ph.D. Others prefer low gear—they make it their business to select a good practice and stay informed, but don't want to get mired in the technical details. I have to admit scenario B was more my speed and it worked pretty well. Still, whenever I'd encounter a waiting-room maven—you know the superorganized breed that have their FSH, LH, and estradiol levels all memorized—I'd feel really intimidated. Then I'd run home, fire up the computer, and conduct research until my head felt like it would explode from an information overload. The truth is some women have a knack and need to learn *everything* and others don't. So figure out which style you're comfortable with and stick to it. Obviously, you need to be somewhat knowledgeable to be a good advocate for yourself. But don't feel guilty if you aren't spitting out arcane IVF data 24/7. You may simply have a different coping style. Besides, this stuff *is* complicated. It takes REs years to learn it. Hopefully, you'll achieve your goal long before you've mastered every infertility acronym and ten-dollar term. (Then, you won't need them anymore.)

And while we're on the subject of guilt I'd like to close this chapter with a final thought: Let yourself off the hook for those times you're feeling less than positive. One of the most painful issues IVFers grapple with is the sense that maybe they're responsible for their infertility problems because they're simply not hopeful enough. It's easy to fall into a trap, thinking: *If only I was more positive, if only I was more optimistic, then I would have a baby now.* This was certainly the case for Shari, a 36-year-old chef: "After my IVF cycle failed, I felt really hopeless. My doctor told me I had a good chance if I tried again, but I just couldn't get out of my funk. Then, on top of everything else, I started to worry that I was jinxing the process with my bad vibes." The epilogue to her story? She just gave birth to a baby girl following her second attempt at IVF.

Sure, a positive outlook is a great tool. No doubt it will help you get through the process with greater ease. But the fact is that a negative mind-set, in and of itself, won't affect the outcome of an IVF cycle. In vitro is a highly technical and scientific procedure. Remember: A sperm gets united with an egg in a lab dish, then the resulting embryo is injected into your uterus. Does this sound like a process that could be influenced by bad vibes? Shari was pretty tense during her second round of IVF—as was I—and science worked for both of us despite our trepidation.

So don't give those feelings of hopelessness too much credence. If they come around, remind yourself they are just thoughts. Just air. They are not fact. Not truth. The only way negative thinking can impact your treatment is if you give up prematurely. So put one foot in front of the other and concentrate on doing the right things to get the job done. That constructive act may make you start to feel better already.

Chapter 5

Funding Your Fertility Treatments

ॐ

The Chance for a Baby, but at What Cost?

Ever go shopping for a new car? If you're anything like me, that five-digit number stuck to the side window is enough to give you heart palpitations. After a while, though, you calm down and grudgingly make peace with it. Then come the extras. Sure, you can forgo the genuine leather seats and club-worthy sound system, but what about the power steering, air conditioning, and alarm system? In truth, they're essentials. They'll also add plenty to the price tag. That means you'll end up parting with a lot more cash than you had originally planned.

Unfortunately, the same thing happens with IVF. A standard cycle runs between $6,000 and $10,000. Then—as if that's not expensive enough—you have to cover the cost of medication ($2,000 to $4,000), anesthesia ($400 to $750), and the cryopreservation of extra embryos ($500 to $1,200 a year). If you're grappling with male factor, it's likely you'll require ICSI to ensure fertilization ($750 to $2,500), and if you're relying on donor eggs, expect to spend another $5,000 to $15,000. My point? When all is said and done, the IVF figure you banked on can balloon to $10,000, $15,000, $25,000, or more. (For a complete menu of procedures and prices see page 86.)

Mark Twain said, "If you have to swallow a frog, do it first thing in the morning." I decided to follow his lead and begin this chapter with a frustrating fact: IVF is a pricey proposition. Why? The process requires state-of-the-art equipment, costly medications, around-the-clock monitoring, and a top-notch staff of doctors, nurses, and meticulously trained embryologists. Plus, people are *actually willing* to pay these exorbitant rates.

"Just tell a woman she can't have a baby and she'll move heaven and earth to make it happen," confirms Elizabeth, a 32-year-old artist currently saving toward IVF. "How do you put a price tag on a child?" How indeed? The value of a new car is quantifiable, the chance to have a baby is not.

But how on earth do people pull together the resources to pay for such a costly endeavor? Don't despair. With careful planning and a healthy dose of creativity, in vitro fertilization is likely within reach. This chapter will help make it more affordable by showing you how to maximize your insurance coverage, tap existing sources of cash, and take advantage of a new breed of "shared-risk" payment plans. It's my hope that these proven strategies will enable you to bring home a baby without breaking the bank.

The IVF Menu

Following are the range of prices you can expect to pay for a single cycle of IVF.

Cost of Total Treatment for a Standard Cycle: $8,000 to $20,000

Here's the Breakdown:

IVF Cycle: **$5,000 to $10,000**
(This usually includes ultrasound monitoring,
standard bloodwork, egg retrieval, embryo
transfer, culture and fertilization, standard
sperm prep, and management fees)

Initial Consultation: **$200 to $500**

Screening Tests: **$500 to $5,000**

The IVF Menu *(continued)*

Medications:	**$2,000 to $4,000**
Anesthesia for Egg Retrieval:	**$400 to $750**

Extras:

Intracytoplasmic Sperm Injection (ICSI): (When the quality of sperm is poor)	**$750 to $2,500**
Sperm Aspiration: (When sperm must be extracted from the epididymis or testicles)	**$800 to $3,000**
Assisted Hatching: (When embryos are "thinned" to aid implantation)	**$500 to $2,000**
Preimplantation Genetic Diagnosis: (When embryos must be evaluated to rule out chromosomal abnormalities)	**$2,500 to $5,000**
Embryo Cryopreservation: (When extra embryos are frozen and stored)	**$500 to $1,200 a year**

More Options:

Frozen Embryo Cycle: (When frozen embryos from a previous cycle are used)	**$1,600 to $4,000**
Exclusive Donor-Egg Cycle: (When eggs are harvested from one donor for a single recipient)	**$16,000 to $30,000**
Shared Donor-Egg Cycle: (When eggs are harvested from one donor and split between two recipients)	**$12,000 to $16,000**
Gestational Surrogate Cycle: (When a surrogate mother is used, either with or without donor eggs)	**$25,000 to $75,000**

Uncovering Your
Insurance Coverage

After deciding to pursue IVF, your first course of action should be to find out what—if anything—will be picked up by your insurance company. Insurance coverage varies widely, with benefits ranging from excellent (a $100,000 lifetime cap to use at any practice), to so-so (reimbursement for specific components of your treatment), to lousy (the big goose egg). How do you find out which category you fall into? By channeling your inner detective and summoning forth every ounce of your sleuthing abilities. Why? The terminology contained in insurance contracts is so cagey it may seem like it's written in code. And with good reason on the part of the insurer. Think about it: If we throw up our hands and walk away, they save themselves a heck of a lot of cash. After all, it might just be easier to fund IVF ourselves than to spend one more minute navigating the legalese of our insurance contract or being put on hold by a not-so-eager-to-please customer service rep. Right?

Wrong! Don't let frustration force you into lethargy. True, less than 20 percent of those who pursue IVF are substantially covered. But you could be one of them! Great benefits crop up in unlikely places, such as policies maintained by the government, trade unions, or a surprisingly benevolent employer. Plus, you may be in a position to take advantage of a slew of recent legislation requiring certain companies in certain states to pay for IVF.

But even if you find that you're not entitled to a global benefit, it's still quite possible that you will be covered for *some aspect* of your treatment, including diagnosis, blood work and ultrasound, or medication. Careful research enabled me to shave about $3,000—the cost of medication—off the price of each cycle. And, unless you're a celebrity IVFer like Celine Dion, that's not chump change. So take the time to get the facts on your policy. This section will walk you through the steps involved in uncovering your actual coverage. First, here's a quick 101 on state-mandated insurance.

The Truth About
State-Mandated Insurance

Currently, only fifteen states have passed laws concerning infertility benefits. In twelve of them—Arkansas, Hawaii, Illinois, Louisiana, Maryland, Massachusetts, Montana, Ohio, New Jersey, New York, Rhode Island, and West Virginia—insurance companies are required *to provide* some level of insurance coverage for infertility or IVF. That varies from the best-case scenario, such as Massachusetts, where up to four in-vitro cycles are covered, to Ohio, where *some* treatments related to infertility are covered, but not specifically IVF. In the remaining three states with existing law—California, Connecticut, and Texas—insurance companies are only required *to offer* infertility or IVF coverage to employers, who then have the option of choosing whether or not to purchase it for their employees. Sadly, most choose the latter.

Unfortunately, there's another big catch that leaves many potential IVFers in all of these states out in the cold. If you work for a company that is "self-insured," as most large companies with more than 500 employees are, the state mandates simply don't apply. Why? Because these larger companies are beholden to *federal* insurance mandates— and, at present, there aren't any federal mandates pertaining to infertility. That means if you live in one of these states and your employer is self-insured you won't be eligible for these carefully crafted policies even if you stand on your head. But don't throw in the towel. Infertility legislation is a crazy quilt of quirky state-by-state policy. It's also a moving target with new laws being added to the books each year, thanks in large part to dedicated lobbying groups like Resolve and the American Infertility Association. They're fighting to get everyone covered and are making some headway. Therefore, no matter where you live, be sure to get all the facts on coverage in your state. Who knows? Maybe you'll be the beneficiary of existing policy or a brand new law.

For a thumbnail review of current legislation, take a look at the table entitled Fast Facts on State-Mandated Insurance. But don't stop there. Confirm the extent of your benefits—including pesky restrictions—by contacting your state insurance commission, human resources department (if appropriate), or your IVF practice's billing office.

Fast Facts on State-Mandated Insurance

Here's a quick rundown on the coverage in the fifteen states that have passed laws regarding infertility.

STATE	MANDATE	TERMS
Arkansas	to cover	Requires employers that are not self-insured to cover up to $15,000 of IVF treatments. HMOs are exempt.
Hawaii	to cover	Requires employers that are not self-insured to provide one cycle of IVF. Candidates must prove five years of infertility.
Illinois	to cover	Requires employers that are not self-insured to cover up to four cycles of IVF. Group policies with 25 or fewer employees are exempt.
Louisiana	to cover	Requires employers that are not self-insured to cover some infertility treatments, but not IVF.
Maryland	to cover	Requires employers that are not self-insured to cover up to $100,000 of IVF treatments, but there are several restrictions. HMOs and group policies with 50 or fewer employees are exempt.
Massachusetts	to cover	Requires employers that are not self-insured to provide comprehensive IVF coverage.
Montana	to cover	Requires HMOs to cover some infertility treatments, but not IVF.
New Jersey	to cover	Requires employers that are not self-insured to cover up to four cycles of IVF. Group policies with 50 or fewer employees are exempt.
New York	to cover	Requires employers that are not self-insured to cover some infertility treatments, but not specifically IVF.

Fast Facts on State-Mandated Insurance *(continued)*		
Ohio	to cover	Requires HMOs to cover infertility treatments, but not specifically IVF.
Rhode Island	to cover	Requires employers that are not self-insured to cover IVF treatments. Candidates may be responsible for a 20 percent copay.
West Virginia	to cover	Requires HMOs to cover infertility treatments, but not specifically IVF.
California	to offer	Requires insurers to offer infertility benefits to employers, but not IVF.
Connecticut	to offer	Requires insurers to offer infertility benefits to employers, including IVF.
Texas	to offer	Requires insurers to offer infertility benefits, including IVF.

When It Comes to Insurance, Don't Assume

After you've explored the possibility of taking advantage of state mandates, it's time to examine your own policy to uncover any and all benefits related to IVF. Unfortunately, this can be a big task. Let me illustrate with my own story. At the time I was pursuing IVF, I worked for a large publishing house in Manhattan. Because I reside in New York that meant no state-mandated in-vitro coverage. However, there was some encouraging news: I heard through the office grapevine that my point-of-service plan included a $10,000 one-time IVF benefit—a bona fide windfall! That coverage was confirmed in my employer's insurance contract with the single stipulation that I choose a practice in network. Not a problem, I thought. After all, there were about a dozen highly regarded fertility clinics in the metro area. Problem was, when I began shopping around, I found that none of them accepted my insurance. In fact, I was hard-pressed to find any practices that would take it at all!

In frustration, I discreetly phoned a friend in human resources. She was sympathetic and offered to do some digging to find out which practices *would* cover me. A few days later, she called back with the names of three obscure endocrinologists. When I researched them, I found that only one had any sort of track record in IVF—and he'd done only a handful of cycles resulting in a single live birth. I suppose I could have gone to him and taken my chances, but I worried about spending the time and energy on a doctor with such a dismal success rate. I wasn't getting any younger. My decision: Take a pass and fund my own treatments with a top doctor. Poof! Just like that, the touted benefit went up in smoke. The moral of my story? Don't assume.

- Don't assume that if you have coverage for IVF, the practice of your choice will actually take it. Unfortunately, many of the best ones are in a position to just say no.

- Don't assume that you are covered for IVF because a friend with the same insurance—but who happens to work for a different company—received benefits. Infertility benefits are purchased by employers as a separate rider and most choose to forgo it.

- Don't assume that IVF coverage remains constant year after year. Companies have the option of adding or deleting benefits at the drop of a hat. And they often do, especially during tough economic times.

Likewise, don't assume the worst. Don't let inertia or other people's negative experiences stand in the way of your due diligence. You owe it to yourself to carefully assess your IVF coverage. Keep an open mind. You may even be pleasantly surprised with what you learn. Let me illustrate with this story of a coworker. Lucy, a 30-year-old marketing rep, had the same insurance policy as I did, but pursued IVF a year later. Over the course of that year, a fortunate thing happened—a new fertility clinic was added to that list of in-network providers. Lucy, a meticulous researcher, turned it up. True, this practice was relatively new, but it was also well regarded with wonderful success rates—65 percent for her age group! Sound pretty good? It was. The only sticky point was that the practice was located in Stamford, Connecticut, and Lucy lived in Brooklyn, New York.

Could she make the 50-mile trek several times a week to pursue treatment and still manage her job? To save $10,000—you bet. Each morning, Lucy and her husband Dave boarded a train for Stamford at 5:30 A.M., arrived at the clinic by 7:00, got her treatments, then turned around and made it to work by 9:00. "It wasn't easy," admits Lucy. "It was totally stressful. But my husband was by my side every step of the way, and we made it work." Work indeed; Lucy and Dave are now the proud parents of twin boys. The moral of their story? Do your research. It may be possible to uncover a creative solution to your financial predicament.

Fertility Fact: Less than 20 percent of all IVF patients have substantial coverage.

OK, so now I've made the point that you can't assume anything about insurance—bad or good. It's time to gather all the facts on your own policy. But how, exactly, do you do that? What follows is a crash course on the steps to take.

Eight Steps to Establishing Maximum Coverage

1. Consider enlisting the help of your human resources representative. In your quest to pinpoint benefits, an HR person can prove to be an invaluable ally. He or she can help figure out the details of your coverage and even act as an advocate of sorts. Should you confide in one? That's a determination only you can make. If your corporate culture is kill or be killed, the answer is probably no. That is, unless you want the epicenter of the organization for which you work to know you are planning to do in vitro and hopefully have a baby. (Hmmm—excess stress, time off for treatments, and maternity leave if all goes well may not exactly be music to their ears.) If you worry that the pursuit of IVF will be held against you, keep your agenda hush-hush and collect the facts without getting specific. If, however, you work in an open and female-friendly organization—as I did—consider enlisting the aid of a compassionate HR "buddy." Many will be more than happy to perform a genuine good deed for a fellow staffer.

2. Get a copy of your company's insurance contract.

Remember that nice little booklet they handed you on your first day on the job that explained your health insurance? That's your summary of benefits. Peruse an up-to-date copy for information regarding infertility treatments and IVF, but don't stop there. A summary of benefits is often rife with inaccurate information and is not legally binding. For that reason, you should check your company's *actual insurance contract.* Your HR department should have a copy of this on hand and is legally obligated to provide you with access to it. Request to see it in a polite but firm manner. (They don't need to know why.) If you are married and have separate insurance from your husband, make sure he investigates his policy as well. If his benefits turn out to be superior to yours, it may be possible for you to switch to his coverage. Or, at the very least, he may be able to get procedures related to his treatment covered, such as the cost of a semen analysis.

3. Determine coverage based on your company's insurance contract.

Once you get your hands on your company's insurance contract, check the date to make sure it hasn't expired. Then, look at the section that describes exclusions and procedures not covered under your plan. Infertility services—and specifically IVF—are often excluded from coverage. No mention of an exclusion is an auspicious sign. Next, peruse the section that deals with limits of coverage. Read it carefully to see if it spells out lifetime caps for infertility treatment—these typically run anywhere from $1,000 to $50,000—as well as other limitations. It's fairly common, for example, to be covered for the diagnosis of infertility, but not treatment. That means you'll be able to recoup the costs associated with figuring out why you're infertile, but not the actual IVF process. If possible, spend a lunch hour photocopying the document (or at least the relevant pages) so you can keep your own copy. Then, take it home to review with your partner. Or better yet, call in the big guns—a lawyer who's a friend or family member—to help you wade through the legalese.

4. Confirm coverage through your insurance company.

After you've read the contract, and think you understand it, it's time to go straight to the horse's mouth—your insurance company. Dialing their toll-free number and speaking off the cuff to whomever answers the phone—after being put on hold for 45 minutes, of course—is one option. But not a very reliable one. Likely, you'll hang up more confused than when you began. For that reason, it's wise to have a solid game plan in place before making that call. Tom, a 34-year-old magazine writer, relied on the tools of his trade to gather the hard facts. "When my wife was doing IVF, she put me in charge of confirming coverage," he remembers. "I relied on the three P's—I was prepared, patient, and pleasant. My questions were written down in a reporter's notebook so I wouldn't forget them. When I reached the insurance company, I calmly asked to speak to a manager—deducing that a senior staff member would really know her stuff. She did. And I dutifully jotted down every word she said, being sure to thank her for being so thorough. Then I asked how to go about getting the coverage confirmed in a formal written statement. (I've learned through my job to rely on multiple sources.) She happily walked me through every step in the process. I even got her private extension so I could call her directly in the future. That really cut through a lot of red tape."

Tom's approach makes a lot of sense—especially the part about confirming coverage. Customer service reps juggle accounts for dozens of companies and often get their facts jumbled. As a result, they frequently utter false statements—such as telling you you're not covered when you actually are, or that you are covered when you're really not. The latter remark, however appealing, is not legally binding. That means you'll still have to foot the bill no matter what they promise in error. Thus, it's a good idea to get a *written predetermination* of your fertility-related benefits. This usually requires submitting a formal request outlining *every component* of your treatment. This may sound tedious. This may sound time-consuming. But it's the very best way to get solid verification. Tap the billing department of your fertility practice to help you prepare the letter by asking them to break down every procedure you require, along with the separate billing codes. This will ensure that you don't end up paying for the elements of your IVF cycle that should be covered, such as diagnosis, blood work, screening, and medication.

5. Zero in on any restrictions to your coverage.

Make sure you do the necessary digging to understand the true parameters of your benefits. You might find, for example, that only a single reproductive endocrinologist in the practice of your choice actually takes your insurance while the rest work with other insurers. That means if another RE is named as your primary physician, your benefits won't apply. Also, beware of the pesky "reasonable and customary charges" clause. What's that? Most insurance companies do research and assign a ceiling price they are willing to pay for any particular service. For example, if the national average for anesthesia is $500, they will *pay only* $500. Thus, if your practice charges $700, you'll be left holding the bag for $200. Who's at risk? Those pursuing treatment at a top-drawer clinic or in big cities, like New York or Los Angeles, where higher prices are the norm. The take-home message here: Work with your insurance company and fertility practice to get the lowdown on your coverage. Failure to do so can cost you thousands.

6. Keep track of all bills related to the cost of your treatment.

Keep careful records. Keep careful records. Keep careful records. I wrote this sentence three times for emphasis. I know writing everything down is totally tedious. It's also totally important. So keep track of all significant IVF-related conversations, whether they're with an HR person, insurance company, or billing office. You think you'll remember what was said, but believe me, two days later it will start to get very fuzzy. Tom kept detailed notes in a reporter's notebook. Kim, a 40-year-old office manager, took it one step further. "I designed a computer spreadsheet and input everything related to my treatment. It gave me facts at my fingertips. In the end, three cycles of IVF cost me only $4,000 out-of-pocket!" In addition, make copies of each and every medical bill you've paid during the course of the year, whether related to IVF or something else. Why? If they total more than 7.5 percent of your adjusted gross income, you'll be eligible for a sizable tax deduction. (For more on that see page 102.)

7. Submit every claim to your insurance company.

It's worthwhile to take the time to submit every IVF claim, *even those you're convinced will not be covered.* You've got nothing to lose and you may be pleasantly surprised by the outcome. If possible, rely on the billing office of your IVF practice to aid you in maximizing your coverage. How can they help? If your plan covers only certain components of your treatment, ask them to prepare statements broken down by service and, if appropriate, to leave off any mention of in vitro. That's what Melanie did. This 39-year-old realtor's insurance covered superovulatory drugs for infertility treatments such as IUI, but not superovulatory drugs for IVF. Thus, when she submitted a bill for the drugs without any mention of in vitro—voila!—they covered the $2,500 cost! I'm not advocating insurance fraud, but I am advocating putting the best possible spin on your claims. After all, this stuff is expensive. There is one caveat, however: Insurance companies have the legal right to reclaim any payments they made up to three years after the fact. Therefore, if you receive a questionable windfall, it's wise to wait out that time period before you spend it.

8. Don't take no for an answer until it's time to take no for an answer.

Insurance companies have been known to decline perfectly acceptable claims again and again in an attempt to frustrate people to the point of simply giving up. And a lot of folks do. Resist that temptation until you're convinced that you have no right to your claim. If, however, you feel your request is consistent with the terms of your insurance contract, get the reason for their denial in writing. Then, if it doesn't wash, find out what steps are required to file a formal appeal. Do so quickly, as most insurers require your rebuttal within a few weeks. In contrast, expect them to drag the process out on their end—an appeal can take 60 days or longer to rule on. Still, it's well worth pursuing if you think you are right. Fact: Sometimes patients win. And for those who don't, they have the option of hiring an insurance litigator and getting back into the ring. Of course, this is an expensive and labor-intensive endeavor, so it's important to weigh the cost/benefit of getting embroiled in a lawsuit when your actual goal is to have a baby.

Tips on Changing Insurance, Extending Benefits, and Switching Jobs to Maximize Coverage

OK, so far the discussion has focused primarily on getting the most out of your current medical insurance. What about the possibility of acquiring *new* insurance? After all, many of us have access to a number of seemingly sexy plans through our place of employment. I encourage you to check out every available option—you may be able to upgrade! It's just too bad we can't turn back the clock a bit. Eight years ago, AETNA, one of the largest insurance companies in the land, routinely offered excellent coverage for in vitro fertilization. The benefit was so appealing, in fact, that a number of women jumped to the carrier to claim it. Unfortunately, those golden days are gone. In 1998, head honchos at AETNA began to see a bump in enrolled women undergoing IVF—as well as the cost of covering them—and abruptly pulled the plug on the benefit. Too bad. Instead of blazing a trail to make in vitro more accessible, they did just the opposite.

Although recent studies indicate that adding comprehensive infertility treatments to the menu of all health insurance plans would raise each member's premium a mere $20 a year, in these days of corporate belt-tightening that's considered too much. And what about folks who are self-employed and, therefore, responsible for purchasing their own insurance? Are they in a better position to secure coverage? Sadly, few, if any, individual policies include IVF these days. That being said, if you're in the market for a plan, it makes sense to shop around and try to find one that provides some degree of infertility coverage—from diagnosis to medications. To help in your quest, contact an insurance broker or your local chapter of Resolve.

Fertility Fact: A recent study found that if insurance companies chose to cover all infertility benefits—including IVF—the cost to each policyholder would be about $20 a year.

And while we're on the topic of a tight economy, what do you do if you've got great IVF coverage, and then you get laid off? The good news is you have protection. COBRA, an acronym for the oddly named Consolidated Omnibus Budget Reconciliation Act of 1986, is a law that guarantees employees who lose their jobs the right to extend their coverage for up to 18 months, provided they pick up the monthly payments. While this may not sound miraculous, it's nothing short of a godsend for some. Eric, a 31-year-old public relations executive, recalls, "When I was let go in the middle of an in vitro cycle, I freaked out. Then I learned about COBRA. The monthly payments were expensive, but a lot less than paying for IVF out-of-pocket." One rule of thumb: Make sure you act quickly and pay your bills on time—if your insurance lapses, you'll be out of luck.

Now, a word about the advisability of seeking out new employment in an effort to upgrade coverage. Infertility chat rooms are loaded with tales of women who cannily made the move to jobs offering insurance with IVF benefits. But are these just urban legend? No question, it's hard to pull off the old job switcharoo, but it *has* been done. Just ask Ellie. This 34-year-old paralegal told me, "I shopped around for a job that offered great in vitro benefits. When I found one—even though the hours weren't as good—I took it and stayed. Sure, I had to work nights, but almost all of my IVF treatments were covered." Ellie's story ended happily ever after with the birth of a baby girl. If you're considering emulating her example, be sure to proceed with caution. Carefully investigate the new company's IVF benefits *before* you take the plunge and confirm that there are no waiting periods before they kick in.

Making IVF More Affordable

After you've made a careful assessment of what will and won't be covered by insurance, it's time to figure out how you're going to pay the balance. "Affording in vitro was tough," reports Renee, a 36-year-old restaurant manager. "But where there's a will, there's a way." For those without names like Vanderbilt or Rockefeller, coming up with the cash to cover IVF can prove a challenge. Unlike purchasing a car, full payment is usually due up front. Then, there's the reality that you may not succeed the first time around. For that reason, it's wise to try to set aside funding to cover multiple cycles. Of course, that's easier said than done—especially when you're feeling stressed out and less than enthused about the onerous task of turning over every financial stone.

I remember those feelings well. Still, at my husband's request, I dragged myself to the kitchen table for a meeting of the minds. And you know what? Once we got started, it wasn't such an awful exercise. First, we determined the amount of money we'd need for treatment: At the practice of our choice, the price of a single IVF cycle, including ICSI, was $16,000. Since my meds would be covered by insurance, however, I could subtract $3,000. That left us with a $13,000 balance. Multiply that times three and you have $39,000—the true cost of doing three cycles (the number we agreed we'd pursue). Where were we going to get that amount of cash? Together, we jotted down every source we could think of with the rule that we would not edit ourselves. After about a half-hour of brainstorming, our list looked something like this:

1. Tap savings account

2. Use bonus check

3. Borrow against our 401K plan

4. Ask his parents for a loan

5. Ask my parents for a loan

6. Ask our siblings for a loan

7. Take out a second mortgage on our home

8. Cancel our trip to Africa

9. Forgo buying a car

10. Take on extra freelance writing projects

11. Sell Disney stock

12. Sell diamond ring I inherited from my grandmother

13. Have a stoop sale

14. Use credit card

15. Sell Avon

As you can see, the list got more unlikely as it went along. Still, all of these *were* bona fide ways to raise money. After thoughtful consideration, however, we decided to cross off a few items. Using a credit card would mean incurring thousands of dollars in interest alone— scratch that. Having a stoop sale sounded like a lot of work and, truth be told, our junk wasn't going to fetch much on the open market— scratch that. I'd make a lousy Avon lady—scratch that. Our siblings were pretty much struggling to make ends meet themselves—scratch that. Our parents, fortunately, were a different story. Both sides of the family indicated that they wanted to help. Each offered a sizable loan, which we agreed to pay back over a period of five years, interest free.

We were off to a good start. Where else could we turn? Using my bonus check was a no-brainer as was tapping our short-term savings and selling the Disney stock we'd received as a wedding gift. Easy come, easy go. Then there was freelance: A while back, we'd both been offered some pretty lucrative writing assignments outside of work. The time was right to just say yes. Finally, it seemed to make sense to cancel a long-awaited trip to Africa and put off buying a car. A baby was our priority so these extravagances would just have to wait. In the end, our "funding package" was drawn from many sources, but we had enough money to cover at least three cycles. I have to say this IVF nest egg made me feel a lot more secure. If it didn't work the first time, we could try again without losing momentum or having to go through the agony of finding the money for another IVF cycle.

How will you pay for treatments? Sitting down with your partner and making your own list is the obvious starting place. If you're equal parts pragmatic and creative, you might be surprised at the resources you didn't know you have. Additionally, be on the lookout for some other ways to cut corners, such as opening a flexible spending account. Many companies, especially large ones, offer this perk. How does it work? You determine a set amount of your annual income—usually $1,000 to $5,000—to be withheld from your paycheck on a *pretax* basis. Then, that sum gets put into a special account for you to dip into for any and all medical expenses. For example, if you put $3,000 in your account, you'll have $3,000 to spend as opposed to roughly $2,000—the same chunk of your income *after taxes*. Sound painless? It is. The only downside is that you must use the money in the account in that calendar year, or you lose it. Therefore, it is essential to plan ahead and keep close tabs on your balance.

Another way to trim the cost of IVF is to take advantage of a medical tax deduction. Here's the drill: If your annual medical expenses exceed 7.5 percent of your adjusted gross income, you're entitled to write off every excess dollar spent on treatments. Say Trish and Gare have an adjusted gross income of $80,000 and their IVF cycle cost $15,000—bingo!—they qualify. Once they've spent more than $6,000 (or 7.5 percent of their income), every additional dollar (a total of $9,000 in this case) can be deducted on their tax return. Of course, this path requires filing an itemized tax return so be sure to keep careful records of every bill related to IVF—including travel and counseling—as well as any other medical expenditures. (Most of them count, from dental work to laser eye surgery.) And if you're numerically challenged like me, consider enlisting the aid of an accountant. Sure, hiring a pro to do your taxes will cost you a few hundreds bucks, but it could end up saving you thousands down the road.

Five Ways to Make IVF More Affordable

1. Work overtime

2. Take a second job

3. Skip a big vacation

4. Sell some stock

5. Sell a valuable item

Strategies for Borrowing Cash

Now, let's move on to the topic of getting a loan. Paying for treatments by socking away money over time makes a lot of sense for couples in their twenties and early thirties. But what about women 37 and beyond who have to contend with their biological clocks? Waiting several years to save enough cash to bankroll the process could result in their being less fertile when they finally step up to the plate. For that reason, it's wise to have a firm grasp of where to turn for money. Here's a look at the pros and cons of the leading options.

Family and Friends

The most obvious place to go for a loan is a family member or friend. For some, the request goes off without a hitch. When Claire, a 38-year-old hospital administrator, asked her father, a wealthy business owner, for a loan, he insisted on paying for all her treatments gratis— no strings attached. "My dad was the greatest," she says. "I couldn't have done it without him." For others, a favor of this magnitude can open up an uncomfortable can of worms. Krista, a 35-year-old assistant district attorney, recalls: "I called up my sister and broached the idea of borrowing money for IVF. She really wanted to, but her husband didn't. Apparently, this led to some heated arguments between them. In the end, I decided to drop the idea. I didn't want the loan to be hanging over all our heads."

No question, borrowing money from a family member is a tall order—one that can lead to hurt feelings, resentment, and a distressing shift in family dynamics. After all, now you'll *owe* them something. Still, it's often a very sensible solution. If you choose to go this route, it's wise to follow some ground rules. First and foremost, try to pick someone who will be open to the idea and who actually has the money to lend. And prepare yourself for the possibility that they may say no. (It is, after all, their right.) If they agree, hammer out some realistic terms for paying it back. For example, you might make monthly payments for five years, tacking on the prime interest rate. That way, it's a win-win for you both. Finally, don't forget to put your deal in writing and take it seriously. Money borrowed often slips the mind, but money lent is never forgotten.

And what about those lucky situations in which you ask someone for a loan and they turn around and offer it as a gift, as Claire's father did? I say, thank them profusely and don't stand on principle. (A couple can receive $22,000 a year sans gift tax.) Remember, you could really use it. Plus, look at it from their perspective: What better way to spend their money than by helping a deserving couple like you bring children into the world? I know I can't think of a better value.

Home-Equity and Bank Loans

Taking out an official loan from an official lender is a big deal. But so is the price of in vitro. For that reason, home-equity and bank loans are a smart solution for many. First, let's talk about home-equity loans (often referred to as "taking out a second mortgage"). If you're fortunate enough to own your own home, chances are you've accrued a fair amount of equity in it. That puts you in a position to borrow a sizable chuck of change—$10,000, $50,000, or more—against its value, then repay that sum plus interest over the course of several years. The good thing about home-equity loans is they tend to have fairly low interest rates, which, in many cases, are tax deductible. That's right, *tax deductible!* The bad thing is, if you fall behind on your payments, you do risk losing your home. Unfortunately, it happens. Although 98 percent of such loans go smoothly, about 2 percent of borrowers default. Truth time: Home-equity loans are a fabulous source of financing provided you truly understand the terms. If you go this route, be sure to shop around for the very best rates. Also, make sure you can really, really swing the payments. The last thing you need is to sweat losing the roof over your head. (After all, you'll need it if a baby or two will soon be joining you.)

Now, a word about bank loans. These, too, are a viable option for some IVFers. In fact, there are even a few low-interest loans specifically designed to accommodate couples undergoing fertility treatments. If you're thinking of considering one, type the keywords "IVF" and "loans" into a search engine on your computer and see what pops up. Are all of these lenders legit? Most are associated with big banks and completely credible. Still, it makes sense to do careful research to avoid falling prey to the occasional charlatan. And, just like home-equity loans, it's essential to revisit your monthly budget and make certain you'll be able to afford the added expense of the loan. As much as these lenders want to help you, it's important to remember that they *are* businesses. As a result, they won't have patience when it comes to tardy payments, even when excuses are very legitimate.

Borrowing Against Your 401K

Dipping into your retirement savings is a significant step, but for some it's the key to affording IVF. Borrowing from a 401K is a common practice; currently 20 percent of people who hold them have loans. That's because, in many ways, it's a sweet deal: You can borrow half your balance up to a maximum of $50,000. You don't have to worry about qualifying—after all, it's your money—and you'll get the cash quickly. Plus, interest rates tend to be low (usually close to prime) and you have five years to pay the sum back to *yourself*. That's right, instead of a bank, you pay yourself back with interest!

But there's also a serious downside. First, a loan against your 401K slows down the rate of your retirement savings. Second, since you're paying it back via paycheck deductions, your weekly take-home salary is reduced. (Never a fun thing.) Third, and most importantly, if you leave your job, either voluntarily or involuntary, you'll have to repay the entire outstanding balance within 60 days or face the possibility of getting clobbered with a 10 percent early withdrawal penalty and a huge tax bill. Say, for example, you got laid off with a loan of $25,000 outstanding on your 401K. You would get socked with a $2,500 penalty and would owe an additional $10,000, roughly, on your state and local taxes. That's a serious blow to anyone—especially someone who's doing IVF and just been laid off. Bottom line: Borrowing against your 401K can make sense, but it's risky. If you decide on this course, make sure you have a handle on the terms and that your current job is quite secure.

Credit Cards

Last and truly least is the option of putting your treatment on a credit card. Yes, plastic money is pretty tempting. With one smooth glide and a signature, you're golden. But are you really? If you put a $10,000 cycle on a credit card, then take five years to pay it off—with a compounded interest rate of 20 percent—you'll end up forking over a total of nearly $16,000—or $6,000 in interest alone. That

---

Fertility Fact: Prenatal care costs insurance companies about 200 times the amount of fertility treatments.

---

number is in the loan shark zone! Therefore, credit card payment should be a decision of last resort with one notable exception. Randi, a 36-year-old photographer, offers this tip: "I put the total cost of my

IVF cycle on my credit card, earned a bazillion frequent flier miles, then paid it off the day my statement came." Randi's fancy footwork earned her a round-trip ticket to England sans any interest. If you choose to follow her example, however, be very careful to pay off the total cost of your treatments *in full, immediately.* Otherwise those ugly interest rates will offset the perk of the free miles.

And if you absolutely, positively have no choice but to fund your treatments by credit card and make the payments over time, be sure to shop around for a card with the best possible terms. (Available rates range between 8 percent to a whopping 22 percent!) That's a big difference. And watch out for dirty tricks. My brother-in-law has a card with a low 8 percent interest rate, but if he's even one day late with a payment, it jumps to 22 percent on the existing balance and any new purchases! Finally, make certain to check your credit limit before you pursue treatment. We're not talking about the price of a new hat here. The last thing you want is to be declined at the eleventh hour.

The Pros and Cons of
Shared-Risk Payment Plans

Twenty years ago, only a handful of U.S. fertility clinics even offered in vitro fertilization. Today, literally hundreds provide the service and they are vying for your business. Thank you, capitalism. Now IVF practices have to, at least, *start* thinking of ways to bring the pricing down. One novel development is the advent of shared-risk plans. What are they? Although the cost and components of these plans vary from clinic to clinic, they go something like this: Instead of plunking down a payment for a single cycle and scrambling to finance a second if it fails, you purchase a discounted package that covers a total of three (sometimes four) cycles. Then, if you don't succeed in having a baby on your final try, you receive a 50 to 100 percent refund. That's right, 50 to 100 percent! Let's take a look at how single-cycle pricing compares to one of these new shared-risk plans:

Standard Cycles vs. Shared-Risk Plans

Sample Single Cycle	Sample Three-Cycle Shared-Risk Plan
Under age 45 = $8,000*	Under age 35 = $18,500* 35 = $19,500* 36 = $20,500* 37 = $21,500*
Refund = none	**Refund = 80 percent**

Prices don't include screening tests, medication, and special services such as ICSI.

Sound like a scam? Rest assured, it's not. However, there are several "fine-print" issues to consider before you get too excited. First, shared-risk programs cover the basic aspects of IVF, but do not include screening tests, medication, and specialty services such as ICSI. These essentials will tack at least a few thousand dollars onto the cost of each cycle. Then there are the eligibility requirements: At present, most of these plans are available only to women under 37 who meet strict eligibility requirements, including a normal Day-Three FSH, healthy uterus, and minimum number of viable eggs per the baseline sonogram. Still, many, many women do qualify for this type of payment plan. Should they take advantage of it?

The jury's still out, with doctors and patients coming down on both sides of the debate. Detractors feel these plans exploit the most likely-to-succeed candidates and fly in the face of a long-standing medical code: Never tie fees to outcomes. Proponents, however, argue that these packages are a legitimate response to the dearth of insurance available to IVFers. My opinion, for what it's worth, is that they're a good thing. Since you've been reading this book, you're probably quite familiar with my mantra: IVF is a process that often requires three to four rounds to play out. No question, shared-risk plans are a financial gamble. But they do enable couples to maximize their chances of success with multiple rolls of the IVF die. In my mind, it's win-win-win. If you get pregnant in your first or second cycle, you've paid extra, but you'll walk away with your goal—a beautiful baby. If you get pregnant in your third cycle, you save a little money and walk away with your goal—a beautiful baby. And, if you don't get pregnant at all, at least you walk away with a sizable sum to continue to pursue your goal through egg donation or adoption. That's a great head start for a couple committed to parenthood.

So be sure to at least consider a shared-risk plan. These days, about a third of all IVF practices have them on the menu. In fact, some even offer similar packages for women pursuing egg donation. IVF financing, like so many aspects of the science itself, is a moving target. Blink and there's something new on the horizon. For that reason, it's important to do your homework and explore every option before you make a decision. You never know what new deals will be dreamed up.

A Final Word on Funding

"When I learned I'd have to foot the bill for most of my in-vitro treatments, I started to feel pretty sorry for myself. Around me were thousands of women getting pregnant without even trying, *for free!*" remarks Gabby, a 27-year-old special-education teacher. Yes, it's beyond unfair that people struggling with the inability to conceive are hit with the double whammy of having to do IVF *and* worry about funding it. When I got totally down about the astronomical price tag, I reminded myself that at least I was living in an era that granted me a good chance of having a biological child. Just a few decades earlier, women in my shoes didn't have that luxury. I'd take my odds over theirs any day of the week.

No question, affording in vitro is a challenging prospect. However, where there's a will, there's often a way. Taking the time to thoroughly investigate your insurance policy is a crucial step. You may be pleased with what you find out. And even if your benefits turn out to be little to nil, you shouldn't give up. Seventy-five percent of the couples I interviewed for this book didn't have substantial coverage. Still, with diligence and determination, most of them managed to achieve their goal. Some approached their parents for loans. Some borrowed against their 401K plans. Some sold expensive possessions. Some even took the radical step of hopping to a job with better benefits. So steel yourself. Then call a meeting with your mate to figure out a sound strategy for funding your treatments, without breaking the bank. I won't go so far as to say infertility is a blessing, but adversity does breed resourcefulness. Working with your partner to secure financing will likely make you a more able team.

And if you have any energy left over when your mission is complete, consider giving back to the IVF community by taking a few minutes to help fight for global coverage for others. Write or call your congressperson and state representative. Contact Resolve and other groups. See how you can aid in the fight to raise national consciousness about infertility benefits—and the lack thereof. Revolutions don't happen without a groundswell. And nobody knows better than we do that *everyone* deserves the right to have a baby.

Chapter 6

Locating the
Perfect Practice

೩ೀ

Starting Your Search

A few months back, I needed a new dress for a relative's wedding.
What a project! Step one, I paged through a stack of glossy magazines
to get a sense of what was in style. Step two, I chose a price range. Step
three, I browsed what seemed like a million stores, combing through
rack after rack until I finally found the one—a flouncy, knee-length
number with delicate white embroidery at the bodice. Funky, functional, and reasonably priced. No, the dress wasn't for everyone, but it
was *just* right for me. And I have to say, my diligence paid off. I felt
confident during the big event and even received a compliment or
two. (These days, the beloved acquisition hangs in my closet awaiting
a second occasion.) Now, my point: Isn't it ironic that many of us are
perfectly content to spend the better part of a month searching for an
inanimate object like a dress, but seldom do our homework when it
comes to choosing a flesh-and-blood doctor? How did you select your
primary-care physician, for example? Quite possibly, it was all about a
convenient location. Or, perhaps a coworker proffered a glowing endorsement along the lines of "He's not *too* bad."

Ring any bells? I know I spent an entire year traipsing to an ortho-
pedist I pretty much detested because, quite simply, it seemed like a
hassle to switch to another one. When it came to in vitro, however, I

took a very different tack. I decided to take my time and conduct a thorough search. I'm glad I did. The fact of the matter is that IVF clinics are not created equal. Selecting a skilled RE and quality practice can make the difference between having a baby or not. For that reason, it's absolutely essential to do the necessary legwork to locate a great center. That means carefully evaluating success rates, pricing, location, area of expertise, protocols—even the overriding "personality" of the place.

Fertility Fact: The largest fertility practice in the United States is Boston IVF, which performs about 3,500 fresh and frozen cycles annually.

Sound like an overwhelming task? As mentioned earlier, there are more than 400 IVF clinics nationwide—with impressive start-ups being added to the mix every year. Which one should you choose? That's where this chapter comes in. It will show you how to compare practices and locate the optimal one for your individual needs. Read on to learn more.

Doing Your Homework

In your bid to find the very best IVF clinic, the obvious place to begin is with a referral from your existing gynecologist or fertility specialist (if you have one). In theory, a recommendation from your physician is a vote of confidence in a fellow professional. That being said, it's not enough to base a decision on. Why? Some gynecologists are so steeped in the demands of their own practices they may actually know very little about the wide world of in vitro. Plus, what's the back-story on the referral? Is the reproductive endocrinologist (RE) in question a respected colleague with a proven track record of helping previously referred patients, or just a name plucked at random from a generic list of local specialists or some tattered insurance manual? Question your doctor to get a clear sense of whether the endorsement is ringing or rote.

Now, on to an undeniably great source—a friend, family member, even an acquaintance who's actually undergone the process. Ten years ago, crossing paths with such an individual was the statistical equivalent of a snowy egret touching down on the branch outside your kitchen window. Today, however, women with IVF experience are all around us—at work, in our book groups, at the grocery store. And they are excellent resources. If you know someone who's had in vitro, try to gauge whether or not she'd be open to a discussion. If your hunch is yes, delicately broach the topic of her treatments. Where did she go? Was she satisfied? More often than not, in-vitro veterans are ready and willing to share their tales from the trenches. "At the time I was pursuing IVF, I didn't know anyone close to me who'd done it," reports Sybil, a 36-year-old florist. "But a friend of mine had a girlfriend who'd gone through a cycle and had twins, so she made the introduction. When I called her up, she couldn't have been nicer. We chatted for about an hour and she had nothing but praise for the practice she'd been to. Her recommendation carried a lot of weight, especially since she'd been successful."

Getting the scoop from women who have done IVF is almost a rite of passage. If you can't manage to locate any, contact Resolve. This national infertility organization keeps a database of in-vitro clinics across the country and may even be able to put you in phone touch with a seasoned IVFer to walk you through the process. (See *Resources* for contact information.) But don't stop there. No matter how glowing a review a practice gets, no matter how itchy you are to make an appointment, it's wise to dedicate some time to checking them out online *before* making any commitments. Remember the detective work required to get the lowdown on your insurance policy? It's time to play Harriet the Spy again—this time to collect key facts on the practice (or practices) you're considering. The good news is you don't have to leave the comfort of your personal computer screen to do so.

Assessing Clinic Success
Rates at the CDC Web Site

Your first stop should be the Centers for Disease Control and Prevention Web site (www.cdc.gov). The CDC, as it's more commonly known, is the federal agency in charge of protecting the well-being of U.S. citizens. Toward that end, the agency gathers, studies, and disseminates information related to every aspect of health and safety. As you will see when you visit the Web site, it's a veritable cornucopia of facts and figures related to asbestos, botox, chicken pox, infertility, and everything in between. (I have to admit some of the content is pretty fascinating, but try to resist the temptation to read all about the infectious disease du jour and head straight for the reproductive health section at www.cdc.gov/reproductivehealth.)

Once there, you'll want to access the most recent version of a report called the Assisted Reproductive Technology Success Rates. (Expect the date on the latest report to be about two years behind the current date. That's because the data take time to collect.) Click on the document to view its contents. You might even consider downloading the PDF file to your hard drive to turn to whenever you need it. Another option is to print the whole thing out, but I wouldn't recommend it—the publication is over 500 pages long! Thus, it's probably a better idea to print out relevant pages as you go.

So what is this tome, you ask? Think of it as a who's who of in vitro fertilization. In 1992, Congress passed legislation strongly urging all U.S. clinics performing in vitro to submit pertinent information—including per-cycle birth rates—to the CDC each year for review and publication. The intent? To enable consumers like you to make informed, fact-based decisions regarding IVF by comparing real results from hundreds of clinics. Prior to its first publication in 1995, IVFers had little more to go on than their RE's handshake and a smile. "If I could give women doing in vitro one tip," says Daisy, a 34-year-old dance instructor, "I would tell them to make use of the CDC's report. It really became my bible."

How do you use it? First, peruse the opening pages. These provide user-friendly graphs on every aspect of in vitro, from the average age of a candidate to the number of in-vitro twins born during the year. But wait, there's more: The bulk of the document provides "fact snapshots" of every IVF clinic, including the number of cycles each performs annually along with its pregnancy rates, birth rates, and more. While an average person might find such data snooze-inducing, it's invaluable for folks like us. Say, for example, a friend tells you about a particular practice she heard was great. To find out if the place truly has promise, all you have to do is pull up the report, check its stats, and compare those numbers to the competition. Sound like a great tool? It is. What follows is a crash course in getting the most out of this important document:

Six Steps to
Interpreting the CDC Report

1. Scroll through the report until you reach the practice of your choice.
Practices are arranged in alphabetical order by state, with one per page.

2. Check out the practice's live-birth success rates for your age and course of treatment.
Success rates are reported per cycle in these four age groups: *under 35, 35 to 37, 38 to 40,* and *41 to 42.* That's because, statistically speaking, the younger a candidate, the greater her chances of delivering a baby. The odds for a woman under 35 are several percentage points higher than those for women 35 to 37, and so on up the ladder. In addition, it's important to understand that these statistics are reported in three categories—fresh, frozen, and donor-egg cycles. To compare oranges to oranges, find your *age bracket* and *category,* then check out the success rate for *live births.* For example, if you're a *35- to 37-year-old* planning to undergo a *fresh cycle,* the clinic's *live-birth* success rate might be 39 percent per cycle. That's pretty good. (Pregnancy rates, which are also reported and are always significantly higher than live-birth rates, are considered unreliable due to the high incidence of miscarriage.)

3. Get a sense of the practice's size by checking out the number of cycles it performs in a year.

The largest practices perform a thousand or more cycles annually, the medium-sized practices perform several hundred, and the smallest ones perform 50 or fewer. Is bigger always better? Not as long as the clinic's success rates are solid and the resident RE has substantial experience. Experts agree that you should choose a doctor who oversees a minimum of 20 cycles annually.

4. Get a sense of a practice's expertise at designing individual treatment plans by counting the number of canceled cycles.

Canceled cycles usually occur when a woman, after receiving superovulatory medication, does not produce enough high-quality eggs to warrant proceeding to the transfer stage. Canceled cycles, which happen at every practice, are not the end of the road for most IVFers. In fact, they often provide valuable clues that enable doctors to fine-tune their stimulation protocols in future attempts. Still, a high percentage of cancellations can be a red flag that a clinic needs to become more proficient at designing customized treatment plans. Cancellation rates exceeding 25 percent for patients under 37 and 40 percent for patients 38 to 41 are not an auspicious sign.

5. Make sure the practice offers the procedures you require.

Many clinics tout donor-egg programs, but—buyer beware!—some of these have only a handful of donor-egg cycles to their credit. If you think you'll be relying on donor eggs, use the report to locate a practice with a solid track record in this area. Likewise, if you plan on using a gestational carrier, make sure the clinic of your choice offers this special service.

6. Compare the practice's success rates to those of other practices.

After you've pinpointed a practice that looks good, your next step is to see how it stacks up against the competition. This can be achieved by comparing its success rate (for your age group and category) to those of other practices. Live-birth statistics range widely from clinic to clinic. Practice A may have a 48 percent success rate, while Practice B has only a 24 percent success rate. That's a difference worth noting! Your goal is to pick a practice with statistics in the top tier or at least above the national average. (National averages are reported at the front of the CDC report.) Another tip is to compare donor-egg cycle rates, even if you won't be undergoing one yourself. Dr. John Hesla, a knowledgeable RE at the Portland Center for Reproductive Medicine, advises: "Because egg donors tend to be young with healthy eggs, the numbers for women undergoing cycles using donor eggs tend to be consistently high—near 50 percent. If that's not the case, there may be a problem with that clinic's methodology."

Fertility Fact: There are currently 800 board-certified reproductive endocrinologists practicing in the United States.

However, there is a final factor to consider: IVF is not always a level playing field. Some practices boost their success rates by turning away less-than-ideal candidates; others, to their credit, take on a disproportionate number of challenging cases. For that reason, you occasionally find well-respected practices with average numbers. Thus, it's important to look beyond the CDC report. How? By paying a visit to that practice's Web site to learn more about the patients it serves and its philosophy before you make a final decision.

Touring a Practice's Web Site

Ever see the movie *Roshamon?* This 1950 Japanese classic broke new ground by depicting a single event from the point of view of several characters. Needless to say, by the end of the movie you had a lot of different perspectives. Likewise, choosing an IVF clinic requires what I refer to as "the *Roshamon* approach." Before you give the thumbs up (or down) to a practice, it's wise to explore it from multiple vantage points: Get a personal account from a former patient. Collect hard facts from the CDC report. Then, zoom in for details by visiting that practice's personal Web site. Short of a firsthand visit to the facility—

an important step that comes later—the combination of these sources should give you a pretty accurate sense of their services.

Like most sophisticated businesses today, any IVF clinic worth its progesterone has a home in cyberspace. True, a Web site is a high-tech advertisement—so read it with a critical eye—but it's also a window into a practice's character and methodology. Some draw in prospective clients with splashy graphics, heart-tugging testimonials, or chat rooms enabling patients to seek free counsel from a resident RE. Others provide minitutorials on just about every aspect of in-vitro science. All of them tell a story. Use a search engine, such as Yahoo! or Google, to locate a practice's Web site. Then, spend some time tooling around it. First, check to see if up-to-date success rates are posted. Because the CDC report lags two years behind, most practices publish newer numbers on their sites. And—good news!—because of improved protocols, they're almost always higher. In fact, it's not uncommon for a clinic's success rates to leap by 5 percent or more over the intervening period. For that reason, it's wise to try to get the very latest data before making any commitments. (Just make sure that you're cognizant of the type of statistic you're viewing. Web sites often post *pregnancy rates,* which are always significantly higher than live-birth rates because they don't account for miscarriages.)

In addition, try to confirm that the clinic is a member of the Society of Assisted Reproductive Technology, otherwise known as SART. (Most clinics are members.) This branch of the American Medical Association is *the* professional society for doctors and laboratory scientists who work in the IVF industry. Its members hold annual meetings, exchange protocols, and work as a team to set the standard for in-vitro care across the United States. In order to join SART, doctors agree to report their pregnancy data, submit to biannual record reviews and lab inspections, and abide by the guidelines set forth by the society. SART membership is a reassuring sign that an IVF practice has satisfied these rigorous requirements—and is worthy of your consideration.

Next, take the time to thoroughly surf the site and find the answers to key questions such as:

Questions for the Web Site

1. How long has the practice been around?

2. How many doctors are on staff? Are they all board-certified REs? What are the specific credentials of each?

3. Do the doctors see patients individually or as a team?

4. If you have IVF coverage, does the practice accept it?

5. What are the age restrictions? (Most fertility practices have age limits. For a fresh cycle it's usually around 43, and for a donor-egg cycle it's usually around 51.)

6. Does the practice treat women with a diagnosis similar to yours?

7. Is the practice well-versed in frozen cycles? Do they have the technology to cryopreserve embryos?

8. Is the practice well-versed in ICSI and addressing issues related to male factor?

9. Do they have a strong donor-egg and/or surrogacy program?

10. Do they offer Preimplantation Genetic Diagnosis (PGD)?

11. Do they welcome difficult cases?

12. Do they welcome IVFers from out of town?

13. Are they opened-minded regarding the treatment of single women and/or gay couples? (Believe it or not, a smattering of practices won't accept single patients and a number will refuse them the option of donor eggs.)

14. Do they offer counseling services?

15. What is the price list for treatments? What types of payment plans are available?

Getting the answers to these and other essential questions, however tedious, will help to bring the clinic of your choice into sharper focus—enabling you to make a reasoned decision. So take a few hours to gather your facts. Some folks love online research and others would rather dig worms in the garden. If you fall into the latter category, make the fact-finding mission more palatable by turning it into a game: Each answer you retrieve equals one point; ten points earns a bubble bath, a glass of wine, or back massage compliments of your mate. (Corny as it sounds, an incentive like this worked for a computer-phobic friend of mine.) Keep your findings in order by jotting them down in a spiral notebook or print out relevant pages as you go and stow them in a folder. It's surprising how quickly hard facts can get jumbled by an anxious and overloaded mind.

And what about those questions to which you simply can't find the answers? Save those for your first face-to-face meeting with your RE, which—provided you liked what you saw on the Web site—is just around the-corner! If you're not bowled over by your local options, read on to explore the possibility of seeking treatment in other cities.

Traveling for Treatment

Fertility services are not evenly distributed across the states. The truth is most IVF clinics are in populous areas. That explains why New York has more than 30 practices and California is home to nearly 60! It also explains the dearth of centers in the Midwest and the absence of a single clinic in Montana, Wyoming, or Alaska. In years to come, as practices expand their reach with satellite offices, this picture will likely change. But what about the meantime? Just because a couple chooses to live in a gorgeous locale where cattle outnumber people doesn't mean they're immune to fertility problems. Are they simply out of luck? No way. These days, many—if not most—practices are well equipped to accommodate visiting IVFers. In fact, during the course of my treatments in Manhattan, I had the pleasure of meeting several couples from abroad, including a woman hailing all the way from Krakow, Poland! Today, thousands of IVFers' treatment plans include travel. Some folks even *opt* to travel when they don't have to—forgoing the clinic around the corner in favor of a distant practice's expertise in PGD, antibody disorders, donor eggs, or surrogacy. Suffice it to say that your IVF options need not be limited to your own locale.

How does a long-distance relationship work? The first step is to have your records sent to the prospective practice for evaluation. The second step is to book an initial consultation with an RE over the phone. And the third step—provided you like them—is to plan a timetable for treatment. Believe it or not, a two-week stint at an out-of-town clinic is often all that's needed to achieve a healthy pregnancy. That's because, in many cases, it's possible for women to work with a carefully selected local gynecologist for the first phase of treatment (suppression and egg developing), then fly to the IVF practice for the second phase of treatment (egg retrieval, embryo development, and embryo transfer). After that, they can return home for the last phase of treatment (progesterone priming and a pregnancy test).

An IVF clinic set up for visiting patients should be well equipped to aid you in every step of the endeavor—from prescribing your medication, to booking a hotel, to suggesting a few low-impact diversions to entertain you during your downtime. Some IVFers even prefer the out-of-town scenario. Away from the pressures of their jobs and local stresses, they can really relax and focus on the goal at hand: getting pregnant.

If you're considering seeking treatment at an out-of-town IVF clinic, use the tools discussed earlier in the chapter—personal recommendations, the CDC report, the Internet, and Resolve—to identify the very best options. Then, narrow your search to the clinics with the highest success rates, the most reasonable fees, and a history of working with visiting patients. When you find one that looks promising, don't be afraid to give them a good grilling over the phone. This is, after all, a very important decision and you may not get the chance to visit the premises in person before you receive treatment. If you like, you can even ask them to connect you with a former visiting patient to illuminate the experience. And here's one final tip: Save your receipts. Travel and lodging count as medical expenses, and remember, once cumulative costs exceed 7.5 percent of your adjusted gross income, every dollar you spend on treatment becomes tax deductible.

Selecting a
Doctor Within a Practice

Once you've homed in on a practice that holds promise, it's time to pick a doctor within it for your initial consultation. IVF clinics often have two, three, even five REs on staff. Which one should you choose? Personal recommendations from women who've gone through the process are the gold standard. But even if you've got one, it's wise to do a bit more detective work. Here's how: Most practice's Web sites post the bios of REs on their staff. In addition, you can type an RE's name into a search engine, such as Google, to see what pops up. Surf these sources to get a sense of the doctor's credentials. Has he or she been in practice a long time? Published any research papers? Served on the board of a fertility-related society such as SART? All are good signs.

Also, make sure the doctor you're considering is a *board-certified reproductive endocrinologist.* What does that mean? Here goes: On the heels of four years of med school, a board-certified RE does a four-year residency in obstetrics and gynecology, followed by a three-year fellowship in reproductive endocrinology. Training includes microsurgery, laparoscopic surgery, sonograms, and, of course, all aspects of IVF. In addition, he or she is required to conduct substantial research and pass a comprehensive written and oral exam. Board certification—dry as it sounds—is a seal of approval that a doctor is knowledgeable, diligent, and seasoned.

After you've checked out your choices, all things being equal, it's probably best to pick the doctor with the most experience. If you're sold on a particular practice, however, you needn't sweat the choice of one specific RE too obsessively. Here's why: Most of the larger IVF clinics develop a portfolio of effective treatment plans that get implemented by *every* doctor on staff. That means whether you see Dr. A or B or C there, they'll compare notes on your diagnosis and you'll receive the exact same protocol from each of them. Personally, I found that knowledge comforting. The fact that the REs at my practice pooled their expertise to design my course of treatment gave me confidence that I was getting high-quality care.

But it's important to point out that not everyone shares my opinion. Elaine, a 31-year-old nursery-school teacher, had this experience: "I found a top in-vitro clinic and carefully selected one of the REs. And I liked him a lot. The problem was, after that initial consultation, I barely saw him. In fact, my retrieval and transfer were performed by other doctors. The whole staff was good, but I have to say it felt a bit like a factory. I think I would have preferred a single physician who knew my case like the back of his hand." Ah, another case of the incredible disappearing doctor. The truth of the matter is that many large—even medium-size—practices share their patients. That means the RE you carefully picked out may recede into the background as your treatments ramp up.

The upside is that you can benefit from the combined wisdom and experience of several REs. The downside is that you forfeit a personal connection with a single doctor. So here's the take-away: If you're the kind of person who prefers one-on-one attention, it may be best to go with a smaller, more intimate practice. There are plenty of good ones with a single RE who sees a patient through every step of the process. If, however, a large practice and a team approach hold appeal, use the tools at your disposal—recommendations, online bios, and an Internet search engine—to choose the most-credentialed doctor on staff with the knowledge that you may be cared for by several colleagues at the practice.

Setting Up an Initial Consultation

Although your journey to IVF may have begun months—even years—ago, an initial consultation marks the start of your actual treatment and, in a sense, is the first tangible step toward your goal of parenthood. I still remember the day I picked up the phone to book my appointment. As I nervously punched in the seven digits, I wondered if this simple act might alter the course of my life forever. It did. Yes, the process took a while—longer than I would have liked. But that phone call initiated a meeting with an RE who devised a treatment plan that coaxed to life a handful of embryos, which divided and divided, and became my twin sons. It's an understatement to say I'm really glad I didn't wimp out on making the call. If you've zeroed in on a good practice and feel emotionally ready to face the challenge of treatments, it's time to make an appointment for an initial consultation.

And sooner is better than later. Years ago, when I underwent my first round of IVF, I had to wait five long, frustrating months before I could even get in to see the RE of my choice. Today, with so many practices on the scene, doctors' calendars aren't quite as crammed. Still, an opening may not be available for six weeks or more, so don't delay. Not to sound like a broken record, but each day that passes subtly reduces a woman's fertility.

Initial consultations usually include meeting with your potential doctor, receiving an internal exam, taking some tests, *and* crafting a tentative game plan for proceeding with treatment. All of this takes time—usually two to three hours. And although it's not mandatory that your partner be present, it *is* really important. Remember, 40 percent of all fertility issues are related to male factor infertility. If your mate is a no-show, the doctor will have only half the picture, which could stall your diagnosis and the course of treatment. Plus, the event can be emotionally draining and you may need someone to lean on. For that reason, too, it's wise to schedule the appointment on a day that's wide open for both of you. This is not an event to shoehorn in between high-priority meetings back at the office. My advice: Turn off your cell phone, take the day off, and give the visit your undivided attention—*together*.

Preparing for Your Appointment

When you call to schedule your initial consultation, make sure to find out the drill for getting your records sent. Going in cold and reciting your fertility history from memory won't cut it. Your doctor will need documentation. This means a copy of the contents of that fat manila folder at your gynecologist's office (or previous fertility clinic). That also means other relevant medical records. No, I'm not talking about the X-ray of the broken arm you sustained in fourth grade, but I am talking about any records related to conditions that may be impacting your fertility, such as thyroid disease, blood-clotting disorders, colitis, cancer treatments, and pelvic surgeries. If you're not sure whether or not a medical issue is pertinent, pose that question to the IVF clinic and let them decide.

Rest assured, getting records is a bit of a pain. The process usually requires you to send or fax a formal note to the keeper of the records, requesting their release and instructing when and where they should be forwarded. Place a call to the doctor's office to find out the procedure. And don't wait until the last minute. Some OB/GYN practices require two weeks to complete the task (and will charge you ten or fifteen dollars for their trouble). Also, don't leave the transfer to chance. Like socks in dryers, medical records in transit have a funny way of disappearing without a trace. For that reason, it's wise to telephone the IVF clinic to make sure they've arrived *well before your scheduled appointment.* Better yet, consider hand-delivering them. That way, you'll be certain they reach their destination.

After you've crossed the tedious task of forwarding records off your to-do list, it's time to get mentally prepared for your consultation. As mentioned, meeting with an IVF doctor can be an intimidating and an emotionally charged experience. Therefore, it's essential to get your partner on board and for the two of you to truly work as a team. Before your big meeting, for example, it's wise to hatch a plan for capturing need-to-know information. Faith, a 28-year-old grad student, recalls: "I tend to freeze up around doctors. I forget what I want to ask. Then I forget what they tell me. During our initial consultation, Tom was the designated scribe. Sometimes I poke fun at his anal-retentive note-taking, but, in this instance, it really came in handy." Remember magazine-reporter Tom from our insurance discussion? To ensure that he and his wife had their facts straight, he recorded their questions in his trusty notebook the night before. Then, as the meeting progressed, he jotted down the answers one by one. Voila!—when they left the office, there was no confusion about what was said.

While we're on the topic of questions, what ones should you ask? Following is a sample list. Make additions and deletions as you see fit.

Questions for the Doctor

1. *Do you think my partner and I are good candidates for IVF? Do you see any major obstacles to my getting pregnant via IVF?*

2. *Have we overlooked a less invasive treatment that might work?*

3. *What are your most recent live-birth rates for women in my age group and couples with our condition?*

4. *What tests will we need before we begin?*

5. *What type of protocol would you use for someone like me?*

6. *Do you think we might require a special service (such as ICSI, PGD, or an egg donor)?*

7. *When will I be able to begin a cycle? What is the basic timeline?*

8. *Will you be my exclusive doctor or will I see all of the doctors on staff?*

9. *Whom should we call when we have questions?*

10. *What's the ballpark price tag of our total treatments? Are there any "hidden costs" we need to know about?*

After skimming this list, you may be saying to yourself, *ten questions*—I've got a million and one! My advice is to sort your queries into two piles: general procedural questions to try to get answered *be-*

fore the meeting—via the practice's Web site or even your RE's administrative assistant—and specific questions related to your personal treatment plan to get answered *during* the meeting. Time with your RE is precious and you want to spend it wisely. For that reason, it often makes sense to follow his or her lead and save most of your questions for the end of the consultation. Why? Chances are this doctor has met with dozens of other couples, much like yourselves, and is keenly aware of the issues weighing on your minds. If you're lucky, you'll get most of the answers you need—before you even have to ask. But don't walk out the door until all of your queries have been clearly addressed. In my opinion, an RE who leaves you feeling puzzled, pushy, or rushed through the process is simply not doing his or her job.

What to Expect
During Your Consultation

"I remember the day I went in for my initial consultation," recounts Colleen, a 31-year-old speech pathologist. "My palms were sweaty. It was so exciting to be finally seeking actual treatment, but it was scary, too. What was my doctor going to tell me?" The maiden visit to your IVF doctor can stir up a gumbo of emotions, including excitement, impatience, exhilaration, confusion, joy, and—everyone's favorite—anxiety. Make it a point to arrive a bit early as you'll likely be greeted with a pen on a cord and—you guessed it!—a clipboard full of forms to fill out. As I emphasized in previous chapters, don't rush them. Take the time to accurately complete the paperwork. And prepare yourself for some waiting—REs are no different from any other kind of doctor. They're busy, overworked, and often backed up. Finally, if you're not covered by insurance, be sure to bring your checkbook. Consultations generally run $200 to $500, plus additional fees for requisite tests.

In-vitro consultations are usually equal parts doctor meet-and-greet, information exchange, and diagnostic exam. Beyond the waiting room, the first stop is usually your prospective RE's office, where you and your partner will be ushered into twin chairs opposite the physician's desk. Welcome to the intake portion of your visit! A doctor who's taken the time to brief him or herself on your case is—in my opinion—a baseline expectation. A doctor who hasn't even bothered to open your file prior to your meeting is a definite minus; by the same token, one who seems well-versed in your history is a definite plus. As with all things related to fertility, honesty is the best policy. Make sure both you and your mate are completely candid. Your RE can't help you without all the facts. Share any pieces of intelligence, big or small. Also be sure to give him or her ample time to synthesize your case. And keep an open mind. Skillful REs may float a few theories that sound new and surprising. Still, don't discount your own instincts—nobody knows your body better than you do.

After your initial meeting with the doctor, expect an internal exam, cervical cultures, ultrasounds, and the promise of at least a few more tests. (See page 129 for a rundown.) Test-taking requirements vary from practice to practice and can sometimes involve a bit of negotiation. If you're coming from another fertility specialist and have completed the tests in question within the past year, chances are you won't have to repeat most of them. The operative word here is *most.* Many practices are sticklers about key diagnostic tools, such as a Day-Three FSH Test or semen analysis, and will likely require you to take them again to ensure there are no mistakes or lab-to-lab discrepancies. In addition, you can expect a battery of blood tests to rule out a variety of nasty conditions—ranging from hepatitis to STDs—that can interfere with a healthy pregnancy. These tests require several vials of blood, so if you're one of the many who hates having blood drawn, try to prepare yourself in advance for your date with the needle. (For tips, see Chapter 9.)

While we're on this topic of needles, some important advice: Don't drag your feet on routine blood tests or wish them away. It's no question they're a drag, but they're also mandatory. That means if they're not completed by the time your cycle is set to start, it will likely be canceled. This happened to a friend of mine. In the blur of her treatments, a simple test to ensure that she'd been vaccinated for rubella slipped through the cracks and her IVF cycle was abandoned on the very day it was slated to begin. Needless to say, she was not happy to have to do the test, then be placed on a waiting list to cycle. Yes, a good in-vitro clinic will prompt you to complete outstanding tests, but make sure you stay on top of things so there are no unpleasant surprises at the eleventh hour.

Now, for the big question: Following an initial consultation, when will you be able to begin your IVF cycle? That really depends on the nature of your fertility issues. Many of the couples who walk in with a firm understanding of their problem—such as a blocked fallopian tube or low sperm count—actually walk out with a tentative timetable to start IVF. Others will have to be a bit more patient. For them, uncovering their issues will require additional testing—even microsurgery. For those who fall into the latter category, I empathize. It took five months and several more tests before I was given the green light to begin a cycle. Yes, it's hard to be put on hold, but it is sometimes necessary so that your RE can customize a treatment plan that will truly work. Regardless of your scenario, soothe yourself with the knowledge that the process has begun and momentum is on your side. Maybe you can't yet see the light at the end of the tunnel, but you are inside the tunnel and well on your way to your goal of a beautiful baby.

More Testing, Testing

Here's a list of many of the standard tests required by IVF clinics:

For Her

Blood Tests:

- Follicle stimulating hormone (FSH), luteinizing hormone (LH), estradiol

- Prolactin

More Testing, Testing *(continued on next page)*

More Testing, Testing *(continued)*

- Thyroid panel

- Blood type and rhesus (RH) factor

- HIV

- Hepatitis B and C

- Chicken pox immunity

- Rubella (German measles)

- Syphilis

Cultures:

- Pap smear

- Chlamydia and gonorrhea

- Mycoplasma and ureaplasma

Exam:

- Ultrasound

- Hysterosalpingogram

Optional:

- Clomiphene challenge

- Laparoscopy and/or hysteroscopy

- Mammogram (35 or older)

More Testing, Testing *(continued)*

- EKG and chest X-ray (occasionally for women 40 or older)

- Two-Hour Glucose Tolerance Test

- Immunologic tests

For Him

Blood Tests:

- HIV

- Hepatitis B and C

- Syphilis

- Cystic Fibrosis

Semen Analysis:

- Count, motility, morphology

- Antisperm antibodies

Optional:

- Blood type and rhesus (RH) factor

- Tay-Sachs disease (for men of Jewish descent)

- Sickle-cell anemia (for men of African, Indian, and Middle Eastern descent)

- Immunologic tests

Assessing Whether a Practice Is the Right Fit

Following your initial consultation, it's important to remember that the deal is not sealed until you say so. The meeting is rather like a first date with both physician and patient sizing each other up. It's an opportunity for the RE to get a sense of whether he or she can help you; it's an opportunity for you to "try on" the practice to see if it's the right fit. How do you do that? Perhaps the best place to begin is with the doctor. Often, larger clinics require you to work with a team of doctors. Still, the original physician you meet with *is* a representative of that team—so it's important that he or she inspires confidence. Ask yourself the obvious questions: Did the RE you met with have faith that in vitro was a viable option for you? Was the RE candid about your odds for success? Were your opinions greeted with proper respect? And, of course, did you like him or her?

The fact of the matter is some IVF physicians are enormously likable: They have great bedside manners and know just what to say to set couples' minds at ease. Others, however, can be long on cutting-edge know-how and short on the "warm-fuzzies." They might even appear a bit terse. Maybe that's because REs are first and foremost scientists—and they should be. After all, it's research and observation and informed hypotheses that translate into healthy pregnancies, not a winning smile. Don't get me wrong, I like likable people, too. But, if it comes down to a choice between a doctor who's super-nice with so-so success rates and one with a more businesslike demeanor and excellent success rates—I urge you to choose the latter. A year from now, when you're cuddling a baby (or babies as the case may be), the finer points of your RE's temperament will be irrelevant.

OK, time to step down from my soapbox. Statistics aside, it *is* important to have a basic comfort level with your doctor. The patient–RE relationship is a difficult dance. IVF physicians have the benefit of years of specialized training and field experience; we have little more to go on than the facts we collected online and our own gut instincts. Still, couples should feel free to state their opinions and ask any question without the fear of appearing "dumb." They should feel uncensored, unembarrassed, and unrushed. They should feel at ease in their RE's presence. And that ease should extend to the entire practice. For that reason, make it a point to observe your surroundings, asking yourself questions such as: Were the facilities clean and organized? Was the staff efficient, respectful, and friendly? Was the billing department responsive and patient? An IVF practice is the sum of its parts. Likely, you'll spend a lot of time with the nurses and, quite possibly, the billing clerks, too. An upbeat tone around the office is a good indicator that a practice is mindful of the needs of its patients—a very good thing indeed!

Fertility Fact: Less than one-twentieth of all couples who could benefit from IVF actually seek out the treatment.

On the heels of your consultation, sit down with your partner and compare notes on your experience. Did you both have the same impression? Do you both agree that the practice is the right choice? For a final piece of intelligence, consider asking the clinic to put you in touch with a former patient to gain an additional perspective. (Just be aware that you're getting a satisfied customer, not the one that went elsewhere because she was dissatisfied with the care.) If you both agree that everything looks copacetic—congratulations! You've got yourself a practice. If, however, you still have outstanding concerns, keep reading to learn about getting a second opinion.

Seeking a Second Opinion

Getting a second opinion—the mere notion has the power to make some of us pretty queasy. As discussed at the start of this chapter, it's not uncommon for women to roam from boutique to boutique in search of the perfect dress. However, when it comes to doctors, we're overcome with tremendous guilt about comparison shopping. Most folks perceive MDs as authority figures and questioning their judgment can feel impolitic. "Going to see a second doctor felt like cheating on my first one," reports Tara, a 42-year-old customer-service rep. I know exactly what she means, but I found a way to get over it. After all, there was a great deal at stake—namely, tens of thousands of dollars and the opportunity for a baby. In my case, I really liked my RE, but I wasn't so sure about the protocol he suggested. That led me to seek the opinion of a highly respected doctor across town. Turns out the two were pretty good friends. At first, I thought this would make the appointment especially awkward, but the meeting went well. The second RE checked his ego, gave me an exam, carefully reviewed my file, and declared—in his humble opinion—that my first RE's plan made absolute sense. In fact, he'd do exactly the same thing himself. With that, we shook hands and parted ways. Sure, that little encounter cost me about $350, but it bought me immense peace of mind. I returned to my original RE with renewed confidence.

Likewise, Nisa, a 40-year-old art dealer, is very happy she summoned the courage to get a second opinion. "Based on my high FSH and age, my first RE really pushed the idea of a donor egg. In my heart of hearts, though, I wasn't ready to pursue that route. So I decided to see what another doctor thought. Turns out, she believed there was a good chance that I *could* get pregnant with my own eggs. Well, that was all I had to hear. I switched doctors and, fortunately, it took only one cycle to prove her right." Fact: Two REs can have vastly different views on how to treat a patient. I'm not suggesting you dart from RE to RE like an overgrown trick-or-treater until one tells you exactly what you want to hear. But I am suggesting that you resist the temptation to settle down with a doctor with whom you don't feel comfortable.

"I love it when patients leave my office and tell me they're going to seek a second opinion," declares Dr. Nicole Noyes, a respected RE at the New York University Program for IVF in New York City. "I want to make sure they get the best care, too." There you have it—permission, even encouragement, straight from the doctor's mouth. Of course, I don't mean to imply that a second opinion is a requirement. The best-case scenario is that you're utterly content with your current doctor. If, however, you're having some doubts, it's a great option. There are just a few rules of etiquette. First, be sure to inform your original RE about it. (You'll need to have your records forwarded, anyway, so short of some pretty fancy footwork, it would be hard to pull off without his or her knowledge.) Second, share your final decision with both doctors. And if you were dissatisfied with some aspect of your original care, such as an insensitive bedside manner, consider discussing your feelings with the RE in question. Who knows? Maybe that doctor will reflect on the offending behavior and make a change for the better.

Final Thoughts on Picking a Practice

To the casual eye, IVF practices may appear similar. However, when closely scrutinized, you'll find they're as different as apples and oranges . . . and bananas and plums. Some are small and intimate, others huge and bustling. Some rely on tried-and-true treatment plans, others formulate cutting-edge protocols. Which scenario makes sense for you? A sound decision-making strategy can be boiled down to a single sentence: Do your homework and select a program with solid success rates, a seasoned RE, and a comfortable environment. It's really that easy. "I took my time and scoped out a couple of practices," reports Amber, a 41-year-old database manager. "They both had strong numbers. But when I entered the waiting room of choice number two, it was all decided. There was an entire wall plastered with hundreds of baby announcements—most with gushing notes of thanks to the doctors and nurses on the staff. That made me feel good. Knowing a photo of my son, Noah, now hangs among them, makes me feel even better."

Chapter 7

If You Need
Specialized Treatment

ॐ

Many Ways to Make a Baby

A century ago, there was a single path to conception: A couple had sex—sometimes again and again and again—until the woman became pregnant. If she didn't, the source of her infertility remained a sad question mark, and adoption became that couple's best hope for having a family.

My, how things have changed. "Today, sex and reproduction can be two different things," reports Dr. Brad Kolb, a seasoned RE at Huntington Reproductive Center in Pasadena, California. These days, reproduction can begin with an egg and some sperm placed side by side in the romantic confines of a lab dish. A man with no detectable sperm count can become a biological father. A postmenopausal woman can become pregnant with the aid of a donor egg. It's even possible for a single child to have five—count them, five—"parenting partners" who are intimately involved in his or her conception. Here's how:

1. A female donor to provide the egg

2. A male donor to provide the sperm

3. A female surrogate to carry the baby

4. An "intended" mother to raise the baby

5. An "intended" father to raise the baby

True, a scenario like this one is a rarity and requires creativity and resourcefulness on the part of the prospective parents. Plus it's extremely expensive, costing in the vicinity of $50,000. Nevertheless, there *are* a handful of kids—conceived under this unique set of circumstances—joyfully digging in sandboxes across the country.

The fact is that children with loving parents tend to do very well in the world, regardless of how they get their start. While researching this book, I've had the privilege of coming in contact with a diversity of caregivers—married and single, straight and gay, each with a distinct fertility story to tell. Many of them fulfilled their dreams of babies with standard IVF, while others required a more involved protocol that made use of donor eggs, donor sperm, a gestational surrogate, even biopsies of their developing embryos to rule out familial disease. But all of these individuals have something in common: Because they had to work so very hard to achieve parenthood, none take that cherished role for granted. "Getting pregnant wasn't easy. It took three years, several cycles, literally hundreds of shots, and one magical donor egg to finally become a mom," remarked Maria, a 47-year-old restaurant hostess. "And I'd do it over again in a heartbeat. My daughter is the light of my life."

Specialized treatments are sometimes the make-or-break component of the in vitro fertilization process. Maria, for example, would not have been able to conceive without the essential "helping hand" of an egg donor. This chapter focuses on a number of helping hands now available. I'll begin with a crash course on the lesser-known members of the reproductive technology family—namely, GIFT, ZIFT, and TOT—which may prove a viable solution for readers with ethical objections to standard in vitro. I'll then explain the donor-egg process in detail, including tips for managing both the emotional and technical aspects of this increasingly popular protocol. Next, I'll discuss embryo donation, gestational surrogacy, and sperm donation. Last, I'll describe how some folks are making use of Preimplantation

Genetic Diagnosis to rid their blood lines of devastating diseases like hemophilia and sickle-cell anemia.

Fertility Fact: Gamete Intrafallopian Transfer (GIFT) and Zygote Intrafallopian Transfer (ZIFT) account for about 1.5 percent of all assisted reproductive technology cycles performed in the United States.

No question, the high-tech, highly personalized treatments outlined in this chapter are not for everybody. In fact, most IVFers don't need them. But one may prove to be the key to conception for you. "Keep an open mind," advised Maria. "You may be surprised at the lengths you're willing to go to have a healthy baby." Read on to learn more.

The Scoop on ZIFT, GIFT, and TOT

If you've done some homework on in vitro fertilization, chances are you've stumbled across the terms GIFT and ZIFT and wondered what they are, and if you should be considering them. Hence, this crash course. Gamete Intrafallopian Transfer, acronym GIFT, and Zygote Intrafallopian Transfer, acronym ZIFT, account for about 1.5 percent of all assisted reproductive technology cycles (with IVF making up the remaining 98.5 percent). Way back in 1984, when in vitro was still in its infancy with pretty dismal success rates, some West Coast REs made a bit of a splash with a new spin on the process. They dubbed it GIFT and even came up with a nifty slogan—*GIFT gives the gift of life.*

GIFT is similar to IVF with a few notable distinctions. Like IVF, a female undergoing GIFT takes superovulatory medication to stimulate the development of many eggs, which are carefully monitored and then harvested at their peak. Like IVF, the male partner produces a semen sample. But unlike IVF, in which fertilized embryos are placed directly in the uterus, the GIFT process injects a mixture of eggs and sperm into the *fallopian tubes*. This is achieved by laparoscopy while the patient is under general anesthesia. If all goes well, the sperm and eggs form an embryo or two, then make their pilgrimage to the uterus for implantation. ZIFT is a twist on GIFT. In this process, the eggs and sperm are placed together in lab dishes to mate. If and when they do, the newly formed embryos are injected into the fallopian tubes via laparoscopy. Then, these embryos journey to the uterus.

Since GIFT and ZIFT make ample use of the fallopian tubes, they are not a viable option for women with tubal obstructions. (It's also important to note that GIFT is a bad choice when sperm quality is poor.) And here are a few more cons: Because of their reliance on laparoscopy, a surgical procedure, both approaches are slightly riskier than in vitro and often a bit more costly.

Let's see: more expensive, more invasive, and a bit less safe. Why then, you may be asking, would a patient opt for GIFT or ZIFT over IVF? Probably, it has a lot to do with their auspicious beginnings: When these alternatives to in vitro burst on the scene two decades ago, the statistics looked quite promising. Thus, REs clamored to add them to their portfolio of treatments. But while the success rates for IVF have steadily increased over time, GIFT and ZIFT don't seem to be keeping pace. As a result, most doctors have lost interest in them, many dropping the treatments altogether. That being said, a few REs *still believe* that some patients do better when their eggs and sperm— or embryos—are placed in the nurturing environment of the fallopian tubes, which facilitates a more natural journey to the uterus. Also, GIFT (but not ZIFT) offers members of certain religions that oppose lab-dish fertilization a process that doesn't conflict with their moral beliefs.

While we're on the topic of religion, let me slip in a word about Tubal Ovum Transfer, acronym TOT. TOT is a lot like GIFT, except that it was specifically designed to meet the needs of devout Catholics. Although it's estimated that the majority of Catholics personally approve of in vitro—and thousands upon thousands have done it—the Catholic Church officially opposes all assisted reproductive technology, with the exception of TOT. "Tubal Ovum Transfer was developed in 1983 and approved for implementation by theologians of the Catholic Church," states Dr. David McLaughlin, a highly regarded RE at Indianapolis Medical Center. He currently performs a number of TOT cycles each year and reports high success rates. Every step of TOT is carefully correlated with the Church's official stance on sex, masturbation, and contraception. For example, the semen is collected during natural, at-home intercourse between a married couple with the aid of a perforated sheath. (The sheath is perforated to enable a small amount of semen to enter the cervix, theoretically allowing for regular conception.) In addition, the eggs and sperm are whisked directly to the fallopian tubes without screening or genetic manipulations—two practices the Church is against.

Because the union of the sperm and egg are the result of sex between a married couple and because the egg and sperm are fertilized inside the fallopian tubes—à la GIFT—this process meets Vatican-approved guidelines.

Unfortunately, as with GIFT and ZIFT, TOT is not an effective treatment for women with blocked tubes or men with poor-quality sperm. And it's not widely available. If this process sounds like it might be a good solution for you, contact Dr. David McLaughlin (www.reproductivesurgery.yourmd.com) or seek out a practice in your area that might be willing to add TOT to its repertoire. You never know. Some REs have considerable experience meeting the special religious needs of patients.

Exploring the Option of Donor Eggs

Around the same time that GIFT and ZIFT were taking off in the United States, another IVF innovation was under way halfway around the world. And this was a biggie. At a hospital in Melbourne, Australia, the very first baby conceived from a donor egg was born in 1983. REs harvested a healthy egg from a third-party donor, who exited stage left. That egg was then fertilized with the intended mother's husband's sperm and the resulting embryo was implanted in her uterus. Although the newborn wasn't formed from that woman's DNA, she carried the baby, she nurtured the baby, and the baby was hers in every sense of the word.

After that initial triumph, it didn't take REs long to figure out they were on to something. In vitro performed with donor eggs would provide a myriad of women, especially those over 40, a solution to their infertility woes. Although it took some tinkering to streamline the process, donor-egg cycles were a viable option by the mid-1990s and a popular one by the year 2000. To date, tens of thousands of babies have been born via this unique partnership between mother, father, and egg donor. In fact, roughly 11 percent of all IVF cycles make use of third-party eggs and that number is on the rise. Why? The short answer is that it's a highly successful protocol. The national live-birth rate for women undergoing a donor-egg cycle is nearly 47 percent and is as high as 60 or 70 percent at the best practices. That's far above the national average for regular IVF. What's the reason? Egg donors tend to be women in their twenties with eggs that are young, healthy, and plentiful. And, as I've mentioned in previous chapters, egg quality is the number one determinant of in-vitro success. All of this is excellent news for the many women who simply can't get pregnant on their own because of:

- poor egg quality or premature ovarian failure

- absence of one or both ovaries due to surgery

- damage to the ovaries resulting from radiation or chemotherapy

- multiple failed IVF cycles

- age-related infertility

How exactly does the process work? With donor eggs, in vitro fertilization becomes a job share of sorts, with two women teaming up for the essential task of conception. First, the egg donor's ovaries are stimulated with superovulatory medications to produce multiple

eggs. (And usually they do: It's not uncommon for a donor to produce 12 to 40 healthy eggs!) Meanwhile, the recipient—otherwise
known as the "intended mother"—receives daily supplements of estrogen and then progesterone to build up the uterine lining and
prepare her body for pregnancy. When the donor's eggs reach their
peak, they're harvested via a fine needle, combined with the male
partner's sperm in a lab dish, coaxed into embryos, then implanted a
few days later into the waiting womb of the intended mother. (Extra
embryos can be frozen for subsequent cycles.) Often, all of this happens with the two women never meeting face to face, or even knowing each other's names. Time elapsed: a little more than a month, or
the same period of time as a regular round of in vitro.

Fertility Fact: In 2003, a 65-year-old woman in India had a
healthy baby boy thanks to a donor egg. She is the oldest
woman on record to give birth.

For many IVFers, egg donation is truly a godsend because it affords the female partner the unique opportunity to be pregnant and
carry a baby. Still, not everyone is a fan. It's not uncommon for a
woman to find the notion of carrying a child genetically linked to
her partner and a third party—but not her—simply outside her comfort zone. Both viewpoints are valid. Is in vitro with donor eggs the
right choice for you? That huge and highly personal question will be
explored in the next section.

Coming to Terms with
the Idea of an Egg Donor

Polly is a respected 48-year-old literary critic. She is also up to her
elbows in diapers and loving every minute of it. But don't let her
elation trick you into thinking that the birth of her little boy was
easy. The road to this amazing baby, courtesy of an egg donor, was a

decade in the making. For years she tried naturally to have a child, graduating to intrauterine insemination and, when that failed, stepping up to IVF. After three unsuccessful in-vitro cycles, her doctor gingerly delivered the news: In his assessment, her FSH was too high and her eggs were simply too old to merit another try. "Those words were devastating," she recalls. True, he did dangle the idea of a donor, but she just wasn't ready. "I needed to take some time off to get my head straight," she recalls. So she did. She started therapy to cope with the pain of giving up on her vision of a child endowed with her husband's hazel eyes and her own strawberry-blond hair.

Two years later, as if emerging from a cocoon, she and her husband had a new plan: They would pursue an egg donor, but only on their terms. Polly felt strongly that an anonymous donor, while a good option for others, just wasn't for them. Over a bottle of wine, she asked a dear friend if it would be OK to approach her 24-year-old daughter about the possibility of her becoming an egg donor. Long story short: Her friend said "yes" as did the daughter, after much rumination. One year and two donor-egg cycles later, Polly became pregnant with a baby boy. "It's wonderful!" she says. "It might sound kind of Hallmark card-y, but the arrival of our son has made our life complete. This is our happily ever after."

Happy endings notwithstanding, the decision to rely on donor eggs cannot be rushed or coerced. "Coming to terms with egg donation takes time," stresses Carole Lieber Wilkins, a Los Angeles therapist who specializes in fertility issues. "It's important to process your emotions, think your decision through, and grieve the biological child that you will not have." Women can feel depressed, defective, and filled with self-blame. Sandy, a 39-year-old dental assistant, recalls how "I ran, worked out, ate right. And I remember thinking, if only I'd taken better care of my eggs, they'd still be good." Fact: Although every woman's biological clock ticks at a different speed, none has the power to influence the quality of her eggs, positively or negatively. In addition, it's not uncommon for women to feel jealous of their male partners who *will* retain a biological link to the child (provided his sperm is used to fertilize the donor eggs). "I know it sounds kind of crazy, but I was really pissed off—pissed off at the universe and my husband—that I had to be the one who had to give up the genetic bond," recalls Brenda, a 37-year-old stock broker.

As with many other aspects of IVF, emotions related to a donor ovum have a way of running rampant. Being told you can't have a baby imprinted with your own DNA can be tough. True, you may have a child, a wonderful child, but he or she may not immediately correspond with the specific image held for so long in your mind's eye. Revising your dreams can take months or even years. And some will decide donor eggs are just not for them, opting instead to pursue adoption or child-free living. Fortunately, since most donor-egg programs accept women up to the age of 51 (or older), the crushing need to beat the clock is usually not such an issue. Therefore, couples should take the necessary time to make a well-considered, heartfelt decision. In order to do that, it's wise to address some key points. If you're contemplating egg donation, here is a list of questions for you and your mate. Try to set aside some time, when you're both relaxed, to read and discuss them together.

Is Egg Donation Right For Us? Self-Test

1. *Can your personal definition of a parent be expanded to accommodate the use of an egg donor? Does this "helping hand" correspond with your ethics and values?*

2. *Are you comfortable with the idea that your child will be genetically linked to a third party?*

3. *Will you be comfortable with a possibly limited knowledge of your egg donor and, therefore, a limited knowledge of half your child's lineage?*

4. *The use of an egg donor means that the male partner, but not the female partner, will have a genetic connection to the child. Are you fairly certain that this knowledge won't disturb the balance of intimacy and "power" in your relationship?*

5. Do you have the time and energy to commit to this challenging prospect? Do you feel physically ready to deal with a pregnancy?

6. An egg-donor IVF cycle usually costs between $16,000 and $30,000. Do you have the funds to afford it?

7. A large percentage of donor-egg cycles result in multiple births. Have you addressed and planned for this very real possibility?

8. A large percentage of couples who use donor eggs are 45 and beyond. If you fall into this category, are you at peace with the notion of being "older" parents?

9. Can you replace your dream of a biological child with a new "dream baby" created with a donor egg?

10. Have you ruled out adoption or living without children as preferable options?

If you or your partner answered no to any of these questions, that's an indication that you may not be quite ready to pursue egg donation. If this happens, don't despair. Resume your talks in a month or two. For many, the choice to use a donor is a work in progress. It can take several weeks, months, even years to arrive at a final decision.

Locating an Appropriate Egg Donor

If you've made up your mind to pursue egg donation, the next step is to locate the very best donor for your needs. For some, it's a woman they've literally only met on paper. "My IVF practice provided a brief profile including the donor's ethnic background along with her health records," reports Ellen, a 41-year-old event planner. "And to tell you the truth, I really didn't want to know more. I wanted her to be healthy, but anonymous. After all, I was going to be the mom." For others, like Polly, only a donor that they know personally will do—a sister, a cousin, friend, even a friend's daughter. Dyna, a 39-year-old dermatologist, fell between these two extremes: "I'm Greek and I really wanted someone who looked like me and shared my heritage. I live in New York City and during my quest, every woman I passed became a potential donor. Of course, I never worked up the nerve to ask anyone. Finally, my doctor suggested I place an ad in a local Greek newsletter to try to recruit someone. It felt a little extreme, but made total sense."

As these three women's experiences illustrate, locating the perfect egg donor is an individual decision, often fraught with passion and intensity. It's a good thing that several options exist. Let's take a look:

Anonymous Donors via IVF Clinics

Anonymous donors provided by in-vitro clinics are probably the most popular source of donor eggs. Many established clinics, especially those on the East Coast, run their own donor-egg programs, which locally recruit women between the ages of 21 and 32 via advertisements and Web site announcements. The standard compensation is $2,500 to $5,000. Applying to become an egg donor is a bit like applying for a job—only far more involved. Prospective donors fill out extensive paperwork, provide complete medical histories, and undergo drug testing and criminal background checks. In addition, they undergo a series of medical and psychological exams to ensure they're both physically and mentally fit. Wannabe donors with health issues, a family history of disease, mental illness, substance abuse problems, or a sketchy past are simply dismissed. In fact, 25 to 40 percent of all the women who apply don't make the cut.

Who then *does* become a donor? Typically, it's women with open minds and the need for supplemental cash. Some are students or young professionals. Many are stay-at-home wives and mothers. While there is no question that money is a motivating factor, it is not the sole factor. Think about it: These young women are required to give themselves daily injections of hormone-inducing meds, make frequent trips to the IVF clinic for monitoring, and, in a sense, relinquish their bodies for a period of several weeks. Crunch the numbers and you'll find that even those being paid a sum of $5,000 are making little more than the hourly rate at Starbucks. Why then do they do it? Many donors actually have an ulterior motive: To perform a good deed. Some cite a friend or relative with fertility problems as a motivating force. Others simply feel good about doing "something positive." And by and large, the process *is* positive: A recent study conducted by New York University found that 79 percent of donors were satisfied or extremely satisfied with the experience. In fact, many sign on for a second or third cycle.

Getting a donor through an IVF clinic usually entails adding your name to the bottom of a list and waiting—often several months. When your name moves to the top and a candidate with a similar background surfaces, you're contacted and provided with the basics: her ethnic background, height, weight, eye color, and complete medical history. The operative word here is "similar." Clinics will do their best to make a thoughtful match, but are seldom able to cherry-pick attributes that perfectly mimic your lineage. Let's say you're half-Irish and half-Italian; your IVF practice might present you with a potential donor whose background is Swedish and Polish and a quarter Italian. You do, of course, retain the right to say "no" and wait for another candidate. In addition, as previously mentioned, some practices will help you place an advertisement to find a closer match. A Chinese-American woman, for example, might run a classified ad in a few local Chinese publications. While this type of recruitment is often successful, it's not a sure thing.

For those considering the traditional anonymous donor route, it's important to understand that you will never meet or see a photo of your egg donor. In fact, it's unlikely you'll even learn her last name. For some, like Ellen, that's a plus. Yes, she was very grateful to her "mystery woman," but didn't want to be burdened with a mental picture that might bump up against her perception of herself as the true mom. "An unknown donor was the perfect solution for me," she states. Is it for you? If this option holds appeal, be sure to pick an IVF practice with substantial experience and a large pool of donors. And don't be shy about giving them a good grilling about their recruitment and screening methods. If, however, the notion of a totally unknown donor doesn't seem quite right, a donor-egg agency might be a preferable solution.

Semi-Known Donors via Agencies

The sudden boom of in-vitro clinics has been accompanied by a number of cottage industries, including the rise of the donor-egg agency. These expert "egg-brokers," many of which are based in California, have a sole agenda: to match IVFers with their dream donors. Simply type "donor eggs" into any Web browser and watch a myriad of databases pop up—most stocked with photos and bios of dozens of candidates. Some tout models, actresses, Ivy League grads, and MENSA members. Others specialize in nationalities and ethnicities: Greek, Russian, French, African-American, Armenian, Japanese, Chinese, Mexican, and everything in between. Are they on the up and up? Mostly, yes. Donor-egg agencies actively seek candidates through sophisticated nationwide recruitment campaigns including hundreds of ads placed in college newspapers and specialty publications. This allows them to locate a much wider range of donors than IVF programs can.

Working with a donor-egg agency affords IVFers the opportunity to carefully select a donor that meets their personal criteria. Lengthy profiles provide a great deal of information about the donor—right down to her hobbies, the health of her extended family, and her favorite cuisine. In addition, it's possible to view photographs, chat with the donor on the phone, and even visit her in person. Donor agencies aim to please and usually work closely with their clients to meet their specific needs. "I had a couple that wanted to see a snapshot of a prospective donor's ankles," laughs Shelley Smith, who heads up the Donor Egg Program in Los Angeles, one of the largest and most respected agencies in the country. "A rather odd request, but we were able to grant it."

But such specialized service doesn't come cheap. While an IVF cycle with anonymous eggs (obtained from a clinic) usually costs from

$12,000 to $20,000, a donor-egg agency can push the outlay to $25,000, $30,000, or more. Why? In addition to the sizable agency fee and the egg donor's fee (typically $5,000 to $10,000), the intended parents are responsible for the cost of the donor's medical exams, psychological counseling, and screening (including the Minnesota Multiphase Personality Inventory), plus all health insurance and attorney's fees. In addition, travel is often required. Since there are few donor-egg agencies on the East Coast, couples pursuing this scenario often venture to California, which *is* brimming with donor-egg agencies. All of these variables add up to a pricey and involved course of treatment. Still, for some IVFers, it's absolutely worth it. "I've come to terms with the fact that I'll probably have to work with an egg-donor agency," shares Hannah, a 45-year-old biologist. "It was a difficult decision. A lot of my family was lost in the Holocaust and the notion of carrying on my heritage is really important. Since I can't use my own eggs, I really want something close, preferably a Hungarian-Jewish donor."

Fertility Fact: Picture books on the topic of babies born via donor eggs are now available to help parents explain this unique method of conception to their children.

If a donor-egg agency sounds like a solution for you, take the time to pick a reputable one. Start with a recommendation from your own IVF practice and/or Resolve. In addition, do your online research and look for an agency that adheres to the American Society for Reproductive Medicine's guidelines for egg donation. (You can ask if they do.) Adhering to these rules is a strong indication that an agency maintains a high standard of care. And a final caveat: Be wary of women hanging out at fertility Web sites trying to sell their eggs without the help of an agency. While some of these "independent operators" may be legitimate, it's important to understand that there is no safety net of medical and psychological testing in place to ensure they're fit candidates. The best advice I can give is to simply not consider them. "Ovum donation is like blood donation," remarks Shelley

Smith. For some, it's an essential need. But just like blood, there has to be an unbendable screening mechanism in place to ensure everyone's safety. Quality egg-donor agencies and programs administered by IVF practices provide this. If neither of these options seems right, it might make sense to consider a known donor.

Known Donors

For a minority of IVFers, known donors are the only choice. Relying on eggs from an unfamiliar woman, even one that they've met in person, just doesn't feel right. Known donors can be friends or acquaintances. But more often than not, they're family members such as sisters or cousins. Using a blood relative enables the intended mother to retain a familial link to her child and increases the odds that the baby will resemble her. However, becoming a donor is a tall order. IVF clinics require volunteers to submit to a bunch of tests to ensure they're truly prepared for the challenge that lies ahead. By "challenge" I mean dozens of shots, bloating, fatigue, mood swings, and frequent visits to the doctor for monitoring. In addition, donors are legally obligated to relinquish all rights to the child they helped to produce. Nonetheless, it's a sacrifice some are quite willing to make. I was touched when, in the midst of my fertility struggle, a friend stepped forward and generously offered her services as a donor. She had three children, loved them dearly, and viscerally understood my pain. Although it was an option I didn't have to pursue, I'll never forget that selfless act.

If you're considering a known donor, choose carefully. Look for someone who you think will be able to view the special connection she'll have to your child as a positive, not a negative. Candidates should be in good health, with a healthy extended family. And they should be relatively young, preferably between the ages of 21 and 32. In addition, a stable relationship and children of their own are a plus. Why? Experts agree that women who've already had kids will be better able to understand what you are asking of them, both physically and emotionally.

Have someone in mind? When approaching a potential donor, pick a quiet place to introduce the subject and expect her to be utterly flabbergasted. Also, be sure to rehearse a scenario in your head in which she says no, crafting a plan for moving past the awkward moment without resentment. If your potential donor doesn't say no, be prepared to wait several weeks, even months, for an answer. A plea for time "to think it through" is actually a very good sign. Carefully considering the gravity of the request from all angles will help ensure a positive experience for everyone. Fact: It can be a positive experience for everyone. Tammy, a 44-year-old furniture designer, concurs: "My egg donor is in my life so she often stops by to see my son. She clearly cares about him, but understands the parameters: I'm the parent. Still, the baby she helped to create will always have a special place in her heart. Just as there's a special place in my heart for her."

Logistics and Legal Issues

If you're planning to pursue one of these three egg-donor scenarios, choose a practice that's right for the job. Some may have policies against working with agencies or known donors, while others may have next to no experience in the area. Make sure, too, that you explore every option. Who knows? You may stumble upon an off-beat solution that's just right for you. Some IVF centers, for example, offer something called "split donor cycles" in which two sets of intended parents share a single donor's egg harvest—along with the cost of her treatment. The downside of this treatment plan is that it affords each couple fewer eggs. The upside is that it shaves thousands of dollars off the cost.

Another piece of advice: Make sure both you and your partner—in addition to your donor—have received at least some basic counseling from a therapist with experience in egg donation. It's a mandatory step at most in-vitro practices. Use your sessions to work out lingering doubts as well as to design a plan for disclosing the circumstances of conception to your child-to-be. If you think this is putting the cart before the horse, consider this: Experts agree that this key decision must be made *prior* to treatment. Why? Because if you choose *not* to tell your child at all, it's probably wise to keep it from everyone else— even close family. How do you think *you'd feel* if a loose-lipped relative let slip that you were related to a third party and were the last to know? Chances are, pretty blindsided.

So how has the first wave of "egg-donor parents" handled the situation? A recent study reports that 85 percent chose to tell their kids about their lineage (at an appropriate age, of course). Most cited two incentives: One, they felt that keeping the process a secret might send the message that it was shameful, and two, they wanted their children to be aware of their complete familial health history. Makes sense. Some folks, however, have good reasons to keep the process hush-hush—especially those from very conservative or deeply religious families who might frown upon the use of donor eggs.

Last, but certainly not least, make sure you understand and address all the legal issues at the outset. If you choose to go the anonymous-donor route, most practices have standard contracts to be signed by both intended parents and donors. Read everything with care. And while it's not essential to have an attorney read through the paperwork, it's not a bad idea. The use of agencies or known donors is a different story. Both require carefully crafted contracts and the input of a seasoned lawyer. Calling upon your cousin, who happens to be a top-notch real-estate attorney, is like hiring a plumber to fix your car. Fact: Rules of reproductive law are quite complex and require a professional with *direct* experience. Yes, we all love to hate lawyers and we're not fond of their fees either. But thanks to their handiwork—in the form of thorough contracts—both intended parents and egg donors know exactly where they stand. As a result, egg donors rarely, if ever, attempt to claim parental rights. To locate appropriate counsel, get a referral from your IVF clinic or good-old Resolve. Fees generally run $300 to $1,000. But in the context of IVF, that's a small price to pay for peace of mind.

Embryo Donation and Embryo Adoption

Another option for couples who cannot conceive—especially those with male *and* female fertility roadblocks—is the gift of an embryo from another couple. At present, there are roughly 100,000 embryos floating in a state of suspended animation in liquid-nitrogen tanks cooled to −196 degrees Celsius. These are the "extra" embryos of those who've gone though IVF. Many tap into their supply for so-called frozen cycles, but others never use them. And some decide to make them available to other couples in need. Although only a fraction of IVFers donate their embryos, over time that fraction adds up. As a result, there are several thousand frozen embryos awaiting good homes.

Here's how the process works: As with a donor-ovum IVF cycle, the intended mother takes daily injections of estrogen and progesterone to build up her uterine lining, then one or more donated embryos are thawed and implanted in her waiting uterus. The good news is that this treatment plan skips the invasive and expensive steps of ovulation induction and fertilization. The bad news is, because a large percentage of the delicate embryos don't survive the thaw, the success rates hover around 20 percent per cycle. Now, you may be asking yourself, *Why would a woman choose to carry another couple's embryo, when she could pursue the lower-tech option of regular adoption?* One reason is that embryo donation affords the intended mother the special experience of being pregnant and bonding with the baby in utero. In addition, it enables her to protect the developing fetus from exposure to alcohol, drugs, and reckless living. Further, she can take comfort in knowing that the child-to-be is the product of caring donors, who underwent a series of screening tests to rule out HIV, cystic fibrosis, and more. Frozen embryos are made available through two sources:

❧ **Embryo Donation Programs:** Many of the larger IVF clinics maintain "banks" of donor embryos provided by former patients.

❧ **Embryo Adoption Agencies:** These private agencies maintain registries of frozen embryos, then work hard to find each an appropriate home.

While the end product of either embryo source, if all goes well, is a healthy baby, there are some notable distinctions between the two. Programs administered by IVF clinics often provide intended parents with little more to go on than medical records, and broad-strokes descriptions of the donors. (For some, this limited information is appealing.)

Conversely, embryo adoption offers a cornucopia of details. That's because it follows the model of traditional adoption. Intended parents receive lengthy profiles of the donors, see snapshots, exchange letters, and sometimes even meet them face to face. It's important to note, however, that because embryo adoption involves an agency fee and a home study, it's more expensive than standard embryo donation. Nonetheless, some believe the advantages offset that cost. What are they? A personal connection to the donors and an assurance that the match is a good one—with both parties signing off on the deal. Another advantage is that these agencies provide access to literally hundreds of frozen embryos. In theory, this allows for greater precision with regard to synching up the ethnic backgrounds and values of the donor and adoptive families. And, because the embryos are frozen, they can be safely "overnighted" to most clinics in the country.

To date, only a handful of private agencies handle embryos, but expect to see an increase in years to come as more infertile couples became aware of the option. The federal government is certainly onboard. In fact, in the year 2001, President George W. Bush signed a law that provides funding to promote and educate Americans about this unique resource for family building. It also bears mentioning that the most established embryo adoption agency, appropriately named Snowflakes, is an outgrowth of Nightlight Christian Adoptions. Religious affiliation notwithstanding, they are dedicated to placing a diverse collection of embryos with parents of *all* religious backgrounds. To learn more, visit their Web site at www.snowflakes.org.

Like the use of donor eggs, this cutting-edge path to parenthood is not for everyone. And it requires counseling, reflection, and serious discussion between partners. Still, for some, it's the perfect solution. Sasha, a 32-year-old product manager, was devastated when she learned that both she and her husband had severe fertility problems. "For a while we were prepared to live without children," she shares. "Then a doctor mentioned the possibility of embryo adoption, which I didn't even know existed. I won't lie, the idea took some getting used to and lots of back and forth with my husband. But in thinking it through, I realized I really wanted to experience a pregnancy. We're now on a waiting list for an embryo and it's very, very exciting."

Relying on a
Gestational Surrogate

About 1 to 2 percent of all IVF cycles are conducted with the "helping hand" of gestational surrogates. As with egg donors, the relationship between intended mothers and surrogates is like a job share. In this case, however, the roles are reversed. Here, the intended mother (provided she's using her own eggs) receives daily injections of superovulatory medication to stimulate the development of multiple eggs, while the gestational surrogate receives estrogen and progesterone to prepare her uterus for pregnancy. Then, following the egg retrieval and fertilization process, the resulting embryos are whisked into the waiting womb of the surrogate, who will hopefully carry a healthy baby (or babies) to term. Unlike the donor-egg model, in which the donor and intended parents rarely cross paths, the gestational surrogate and intended parents talk and meet frequently, support each other through the delivery, and often establish a lifelong bond. Therefore, it's essential for both parties to have a genuine regard for each other.

Gestational surrogacy is a viable option for a woman who can produce quality eggs but cannot carry a child because:

- her uterus can't sustain a pregnancy

- she has no uterus, but intact ovaries

- she suffers from a chronic disease such as severe diabetes, lupus, cholitis, or rheumatoid arthritis

- she has had several failed IVF cycles

The good news is that gestational surrogacy in conjunction with IVF is a highly effective treatment for a woman with any of these issues, provided she has healthy eggs. (And for those who don't, a fourth-party egg donor is an option.) The bad news is the price tag—$25,000 to a staggering $75,000. Why so steep? The intended parents usually foot the entire bill: in vitro, health insurance, counseling, and lawyers for both parties, plus compensation for the surrogate *and* the agency that located her. In addition, surrogacy can present some frustrating—though not insurmountable—legal issues.

Remember the notorious, headline-grabbing "Baby M" case? If not, let me refresh your memory: In the mid-1980s, William and Elizabeth Stern were unable to have their own baby so they contracted with Mary Beth Whitehead, a homemaker and mother of two, to do it for them. For a fee of $10,000, Mary Beth agreed to become pregnant with William's sperm via artificial insemination, then carry the baby to term for the couple. The only problem was that she ultimately had a change of heart and decided she couldn't part with the child that she carried for nine long months. Long story short: A bitter custody battle ensued, resulting in a 1988 New Jersey Supreme Court ruling granting custody to the Sterns and visitation rights to Whitehead. Further, it deemed surrogacy contracts invalid in the state.

Of course, the "Baby M" case is not legally analogous to the standard IVF–gestational surrogate arrangement in which the surrogate is *not* genetically linked to the child (as Mary Beth was). But it opened a Pandora's box. The case so captured the public's imagination that it became a political hot button. And many state lawmakers rushed to pass legislation to prevent future Baby M predicaments. As a result, the country is presently a patchwork of tough-to-interpret surrogacy policy. Nevertheless, surrogacy *is* legal in all 50 states, but here's the catch: Contracts pertaining to surrogacy are not enforceable in most of them. In addition, it's *not* legal to compensate a surrogate in Arizona, Michigan, New Mexico, New York, Utah, and Washington.

Hmmm . . . that could prove to be a problem. Consider the many IVFers who live in New York, for example. It's OK for them to use a surrogate, but against the law to pay her. That means that unless they have a relative, friend, or saint who's willing to carry the child gratis, they can't legally undergo an IVF cycle with a surrogate there. That's where *other* states, especially surrogate-friendly California, come in. "Yes, people use surrogates in other places. But because payment for them is accepted here, couples fly in from across the country to take advantage of our liberal policy," remarks Karen Synesiou, cofounder of the Center for Surrogate Parenting in Encino, California. Established in 1980, the center is one of the most respected programs in the country and is responsible for nearly 1,000 babies, including high-profile bundles of joy for actor Kelsey Grammar and soap star Deidre Hall. But they are by no means the only players. California is home to several agencies that specialize in matching couples with hired gestational surrogates, and there are also more than 50 IVF practices with substantial experience in the area. (And with pro-surrogacy legislation recently passed in Texas, expect that state to follow California's lead in years to come.)

Fact: The combination of IVF and gestational surrogates has made it possible for thousands of infertile couples to become joyous parents to children who are 100 percent theirs—genetically and spiritually. Despite the memorable Mary Beth Whitehead incident, the relationship between intended parents and surrogates generally works out well with both parties feeling positive about the outcome. In fact, the Organization of Parents Through Surrogacy (acronym OPTS) reports that 99 percent of surrogacy arrangements have been successful. (Lawsuits filed by surrogates trying to keep the baby are the stuff of TV movies and seldom happen in real life.) But this treatment is not for the faint of heart. It's all-consuming, costly, and demands a unique skill set: Parents-to-be must be effective micromanagers, but *not* control freaks. After all, it's only right that the gestational surrogate retains a good deal of the decision-making power.

How does one go about locating a surrogate? There are two basic avenues:

Gestational Surrogates Through Agencies

Locating a great gestational surrogate is a difficult process. For that reason, many rely on special agencies to perform that task for them. "Very few people fit the bill to be surrogate moms," states Karen Synesiou. "After all the screening, we accept only about 10 percent of those who apply." Like egg donors, women who wish to be gestational carriers undergo a great deal of counseling and testing to ensure they're both physically and mentally fit for the job. Most of those who make the cut are middle-class and in stable relationships. All are between the ages of

21 and 40, with children of their own. "A surrogate *must* have children to know what it feels like to be pregnant and to give that child up," says Karen emphatically. This iron-clad rule preselects women who've achieved successful births and deselects those inspired solely by money. Yes, surrogates do receive substantial payment—generally $15,000 to $25,000—but they need to be in it for other reasons. Such as? Surrogates often say that they love being pregnant, feel empathy for infertile women, or want to do something to help others.

Known Gestational Surrogates

Some couples are lucky enough to have an "angel" in their lives—someone willing to incubate their embryos, then exit stage left after a successful delivery. Just as there are those willing to give up a kidney to help a loved one in need, there are those willing to make a sacrifice to turn another woman's dreams of motherhood into a reality. Sometimes people approach a sister or cousin or friend. Occasionally, the potential surrogate makes the first move. "Here I am, in the thick of my fertility problems," says Deliah, a 36-year-old yoga instructor. "I'm not sure if I'll need a surrogate, but a good friend came over one day and announced out of the blue that she wanted to do it. I can't tell you how great that made me feel. If I need to, I will take her up on the offer."

The relationship between gestational surrogate and intended parents is perhaps the most challenging partnership outlined in this chapter. It calls for teamwork and mutual respect. As a result, it's not uncommon for every participant to leave the experience enriched. The intended parents have their long-awaited child; the surrogate has the satisfaction of doing a very good deed. Could the use of a surrogate be your key to conception? Don't dismiss the possibility out of hand. Take the time to discuss this option with your partner, get counseling, and arrive at a reasoned decision.

If you do decide to pursue a gestational surrogate, really, really do your homework. Use the research tools outlined in Chapter 6 to find an IVF practice with considerable experience and, if necessary, a reputable agency to help locate the very best surrogate. Martha, a savvy 43-year-old stage manager, thought she could do it on her own: "To save money, I found my own surrogate on the Web. She seemed great at first, but she didn't take her meds so the whole cycle was a bust. I learned my lesson." Also, hire a lawyer with direct experience in surrogacy to draft a careful agreement. Sure, it might feel a little icky to introduce the "cynical" reality of a multipage contract into your surrogacy arrangement—especially if you're using a loved one—but know that it's an essential step. Most IVF practices won't proceed without them, anyway.

Fertility Fact: People erroneously believe surrogacy is a lawsuit waiting to happen. Over the last 20 years, there have been 8,000 surrogate births and only 12 lawsuits filed.

"With a surrogate there are lots of hoops to jump through," says Mary Cedarblade, an attorney specializing in reproductive law in Fairfax, California. "But the hoops are there for a reason. They help ensure that everyone involved in the process has a voice and an advocate. The surrogacy arrangement is complex. Problems arise when everyone's cards are not on the table," she warns. Finally, make sure you fully understand surrogacy laws in your home state. To learn more about specific legalities, contact the Organization for Parents Through Surrogacy. This respected nonprofit is the country's oldest and largest surrogacy support group. You might just pick up some other tips, too. (See *Resources* for contact information.)

Getting a Sperm Donation

There is evidence that sperm from a third-party donor has been used to achieve pregnancies since the fourteenth century. Back then, it was a key ingredient in a primitive form of artificial insemination. These days, it's sometimes a key ingredient in IVF, too. As discussed earlier in this book, a male partner need only produce a few healthy sperm for in vitro to work. This is possible, in large part, because of the advent of sperm aspiration (the removal of healthy sperm from the epididymis or testicles) along with ICSI (the injection of a single sperm directly into an egg to jumpstart fertilization). But what about men who produce no sperm at all? Or single women or lesbian couples who undergo IVF? They'll all require donor sperm.

As with donor eggs, IVF candidates occasionally rely on sperm supplied by friends or loved ones. But more often than not, they turn to a sperm bank. There are dozens across the country. Many of the larger ones, such as California Cryobank in Los Angeles, enable IVFers to access online databases filled with the profiles of literally hundreds of donors. They can then make a match based on eye color, ethnic background, even the donor's favorite novel, sport, or season. Although photos of donors are a rarity, some sperm banks supply audiotape interviews and/or "aesthetic ratings"—1 is average, 2 is good looking, and 3 is certifiably handsome. (I kid you not!) In all cases, donors' complete medical histories are provided and you can rest assured that their sperm has been carefully screened to rule out HIV, hepatitis, and the like. Who are these mysterious donors? Back in the day, it was generally med students trying to make a few extra bucks. Today there is still a preponderance of doctors—not a bad thing!—but recruitment campaigns have also succeeded in attracting men of every stripe to correspond with the diverse needs of clients.

Lara, a 38-year-old copy chief, shares her story: "Finding a sperm donor was quite a process. My husband and I spent many a night hunched over the computer checking out profiles. It was pretty interesting reading. Finally, we narrowed it down to two guys with advanced degrees, green eyes, and Scottish ancestry (my husband's Scottish). In the end, it was 'blue cheese' by a nose," she says with a laugh. "My husband is oddly passionate about blue cheese so when one of them mentioned that he loved Stilton, we knew we'd found our man!"

In locating a sperm donor, as with many aspects of IVF, it can sometimes feel like you've walked into a theater of the absurd. For that reason, it's important to maintain your sense of humor, just as

Lara did. Be careful, though, not to trivialize the process. There is no question that a double standard seems to exist between ovum and sperm donations. (Remember, a sperm may be tiny—600 times smaller than an egg—but it carries half the genetic responsibility.) IVFers will often go to the ends of the earth to find an A+ egg donor, but are sometimes cavalier about sperm donors. Try not to fall into this thinking trap. Take the time to find the perfect donor for your needs. And if you're pursuing it because your male partner can't provide sperm, don't underestimate the gravity of the situation. Just as a woman who turns to an egg donor must grieve the dream of a biological child she'll never have, so, too, does a man relying on a sperm donor. He'll need your love, understanding, and support. He may even need counseling. So be on the lookout for subtle signs that he may be hurting.

Now, a word about logistics. The cost of donor sperm used in conjunction with IVF runs about $250 to $500, including the cost of shipping it overnight—in a surprisingly large tank of liquid nitrogen—anywhere in the country. If you think you might require third-party sperm, best not to wait until the eleventh hour. Choose a donor well in advance of your treatment and work with your IVF practice to ensure that it gets to its destination on time. If the shipment arrives even a few hours late, your cycle may be blown. And here's a final tip: Purchase and freeze several extra vials from the donor of your choice for possible use down the road. Justine, a 42-year-old tax preparer, did just this: "Three years ago I gave birth to a son using a sperm donor and artificial insemination. At the time, I decided to purchase and store a few extra samples, 'just in case.' Well, as it turns out, my partner Marilyn decided *she* wanted a baby—only she needed IVF. Thankfully we had that sperm. Marilyn is now four months pregnant. And the best part is, our son will have a biological connection to his new sibling!"

Fertility Fact: An estimated 50 percent of miscarriages are the result of chromosomal abnormalities.

The Brave New World of Preimplantation Genetic Diagnosis and Gender Selection

Some aspects of IVF feel utterly futuristic—almost as if they've been ripped from the pages of Aldous Huxley's *Brave New World*. Preimplantation Genetic Diagnosis, acronym PGD, is one of them. What is it exactly? Think of PGD as a very, very, very early checkup for baby-to-be. In simple terms, this technology enables doctors to extract a single cell from a three-day-old embryo and analyze its intricate makeup to check for specific genetic and chromosomal disorders such as Tay-Sachs disease or Down syndrome. If irregularities are present, the embryo is not a candidate for implantation. If, however, the embryo appears to be normal, it gets green-lighted to be transferred to the uterus during IVF.

To test for some conditions, doctors can even start the process a step earlier—by examining an IVFer's eggs *prior* to fertilization! In one recent procedure, Dr. Yuri Verlinsky, a pioneer of PGD at the Reproductive Genetics Institute of Chicago, used this process to help a woman overcome a family history of early-onset Alzheimer's. Her father had died of the disease at 42 and her sister developed it at 38. After examining the patient's eggs, Verlinsky found a single one free of the mutated gene. So he fertilized it with her husband's sperm and transferred it to her uterus. Nine months later, she gave birth to a healthy baby girl and can now rest assured that her daughter will not suffer from the same disease that has so devastated her family tree.

Sound like a promising technology? It is. The very first PGD baby was delivered in 1989. Since then, the process has enabled more than a thousand couples to parent healthy offspring. It's fair to say, however, that PGD is still in its infancy. True, it can be used to test for a host of genetic abnormalities, including cystic fibrosis, Huntington's disease, sickle-cell anemia, hemophilia, Down syndrome, and Tay-Sachs disease. "But that's just the tip of the iceberg," reports Dr. Lawrence Werlin, an RE at Coastal Fertility Medical Center in Irvine, California, and an expert in the area of PGD. "Out of the 23 chromosomes common to men and women, doctors can test 9 of them with PGD." That leaves 14 chromosomes left unchecked. But Werlin predicts that in five or ten years, the technology will exist to check *all* of them, enabling physicians to detect a myriad of gene-related defects—from dyslexia to a predisposition to several types of cancer.

While many consider PGD a modern miracle, some medical ethicists worry that it will lead to an epidemic of "designer" babies engineered to their parents' whims. Some see a day when IVFers will be able to tick off a list of attributes—periwinkle eyes, genius IQ, musical aptitude—thus setting an impossible and arbitrary standard for perfection. Will this come to pass? Your guess is as good as mine. It's a sure bet, however, that the debate will heat up as the technology gets more and more sophisticated. In the meantime, PGD is a great resource for those couples with a familial history of certain gene-related diseases (see list on page 165). "Cystic fibrosis runs in my family," says Jill, a 28-year-old clothing buyer. "I don't want to risk passing it on. I'm gearing up for IVF and PGD will be a part of it."

REs are also beginning to use the process to examine the embryos of women who fail to achieve successful pregnancies—especially those 35 and beyond. As a woman gets older, some of her eggs sustain microscopic chromosomal damage. Consider the statistics on Down syndrome, for example. A 20-year-old has a one in 2,500 chance of having a baby with this condition, while a 40-year-old has a one in 109 chance. In fact, it's estimated that 50 percent of miscarriages are the result of chromosomal disorders. PGD helps doctors to assess the makeup of a woman's embryos to preselect those with the best shot of implanting. And the procedure seems to be working. A recent, albeit small, European study showed that the pregnancy rates of 35- to 45-year-olds who had PGD prior to IVF increased from 16 percent to 30 percent. (Impressive statistics aside, if you're considering the technology because of poor egg quality, be sure to carefully weigh the pros and cons of adding it to your IVF protocol. Most chromosomally damaged embryos simply fail to implant and lower-cost chorionic villus sampling (CVS) and amniocentesis are the more obvious choices to rule out Down syndrome. For these reasons, it often makes sense to simply transfer a larger number of embryos—on the theory that most of them won't thrive—rather than to invest in PGD.)

OK, time to talk cost: Like many of the treatments outlined in this chapter, PGD is pricey. The procedure tacks $2,500 to $5,000 onto the already steep cost of IVF. And since the process is still considered experimental, it's seldom covered by insurance. Another consideration is that PGD sometimes involves travel since only a handful of practices currently offer this rarified service in their own labs. (Two clinics that do are the Institute for Reproductive Medicine and Science of St. Barnabas Medical Center in Livingston, N.J. and the Reproductive Genetics Institute of Chicago.) Therefore, it's imperative to do careful research to locate a practice with significant experience in the field and make sure it's appropriate for your circumstances. The bottom line: When Preimplantation Genetic Diagnosis becomes more advanced and streamlined, it may well be a wise choice for all IVFers. For now, it's a great tool for some—especially those with a familial disease that it can detect.

Preimplantation Genetic Diagnosis can be used to screen out:

- Cystic fibrosis

- Down syndrome

- Early-onset Alzheimer's

- Fragile X syndrome

- Gaucher's disease

- Hemophilia A and B

- Huntington's disease

- Lesch-Nyhan syndrome

Preimplantation Genetic Diagnosis *(continued on next page)*

Preimplantation Genetic Diagnosis *(continued)*

• Muscular dystrophy

• Neurofibromatosis

• Retinitis pigmentosa

• Sickle-cell anemia

• Tay-Sachs disease

• Turner's syndrome

• Certain breast cancer genes

Last but not least, a quick word on a cutting-edge option—gender selection. Believe it or not, as you read this, couples are relying on a state-of-the-art process available from a company called Microsort to preselect the sex of their children. If you've retained a few scraps of high-school biology, you may remember that the male partner always determines the gender of a child. If he contributes an X sex chromosome to the mix, the baby will be a girl; if he contributes a Y sex chromosome, the baby will be a boy. Now technicians at the Genetics and IVF Institute in Fairfax, Virginia, use a machine called a flow cytometer that literally sorts sperm into "that which will beget girls" and "that which will beget boys" with a 90 percent accuracy rate.

You may be unsettled by the prospect of people actually choosing the sex of their unborn children. I know it made me a little queasy at first. Know, however, that there is at least one very legitimate reason to do it. Some men have a family history of disease passed only to male children, such as muscular dystrophy or hemophilia. The Microsort technology enables them to evade the illness by using only the sperm that will result in girls. In addition, a compelling case can be made for using the process for "family balancing." Let's say a couple has several girls, but really wants a boy, too. Instead of trying again and again and again, and stretching their household income to its breaking point, they can pay $3,000 for a near-guarantee of their desired boy. (A couple must have one child of the opposite sex they seek in order to be eligible to make use of Microsort for family balancing.) So far, more than 300 babies have been born via this technology, and no doubt those numbers will increase as more people get comfortable with this postmodern approach to family planning. If you're interested in learning more, visit the Web site at www.microsort.net.

A Final Word on Getting a "Helping Hand"

In this chapter, you've been introduced to a varied group of IVFers—each with a specialized treatment plan. Polly and Luke decided to use an egg donor. Sasha and Mel opted for embryo donation. Justine and Marilyn relied on a sperm donor. Martha and Claus are gearing up for a second round of IVF with a gestational surrogate. Jill and Doug plan on pursuing Preimplantation Genetic Diagnosis. And Samantha and Todd—whom you haven't met—well, they decided to skip straight to adoption.

My point: There are as many paths to parenthood as there are people on the planet. And your notion of the best route may not jibe with anyone else's—not even your former self. "My super-strong will to have a child really surprised me," shares Martha. "It was kind of like an auction in which the bidding went up and up and up. I thought I knew my limit, but I didn't. If you had told me ten years ago that I'd be using a surrogate—not once, but twice!—I would have said no way, that's not me. But now it feels like a good plan. I don't have my baby yet, but I'm working on it."

A thirty-something actress friend, who cherishes her freedom and was always dead set against having kids, called the other day: "I'm having thoughts," she remarked cryptically. "I cannot stop thinking about babies. What's going on?" *3, 2, 1 . . . and so the adventure begins,* I said to myself. The desire to have offspring has a tendency to strike without warning. It is also deeply primal and very personal. One couple's belief system may prohibit them from even considering the intervention of in vitro, while another may be willing to try just about anything to conceive. Is one of the options outlined in this chapter the answer for you? That's a decision only you can make. And it may take some time. So gather all your choices like stones and turn them over, one by one. Then discuss each with your mate or a trusted loved one.

The quest to have children sometimes calls for a combination of creative thinking and resiliency. Needless to say, it's hard to achieve either when you're feeling world-weary. So get the help you need. Seek therapy. Join a support group. Then take comfort in the fact that you're not alone. There are thousands of people who've stood at the same fork in the road, made thoughtful decisions, and moved forward with confidence and success. Fact: The vast majority of women who have failed to conceive eventually achieve the goal of having children with the intervention of fertility treatments, IVF, egg donations, embryo donation, sperm donation, PGD, or adoption. "All told, it took us six years, three IVFs, two surgeries, a sperm donor, and a whole lot of focus to have our twin sons," reports Kate, a 41-year-old photo researcher. "There were certainly times when I wanted to throw in the towel. But I somehow kept going. And now, I'm just a mom—a regular mom, with a great story to tell."

Chapter 8

Gearing Up
for a Great Cycle
ॐ

Preparing for
Your Big Moment

Wow! you might be saying to yourself, *We're finally here, finally ready to talk about the actual IVF cycle.* It may seem surprising that it has taken seven chapters to get to this point. But that's how many things in life are—preparation, preparation, and more preparation before the big event. Ever dabble in theater? I did. In high school I auditioned for *Fiddler on the Roof* and earned a tiny, but coveted, role as a bottle dancer. The play was my first and I remember being struck by just how much work went into it. Costumes had to be sewn. Money had to be raised to pay for sets. And, of course, the actors had to learn their lines. All of this took time, but our dedication paid off. On the night of the performance, we knew just what to do.

IVF is similar. There is so much to take care of *before* a cycle starts—undergoing tests, finding funding, locating a practice—that it's natural for IVFers to arrive at their start date excited and a little stressed out. "When our RE finally gave me the go-ahead to begin in vitro, it was kind of surreal," remarks Noelle, a 30-year-old bookkeeper. "My husband and I planned and saved and talked about it for so long, I literally had butterflies!" No question, when the curtain rises on your actual cycle, you may find yourself in a state very similar to opening night jitters. I remember how I felt: I was worried about the medical procedures. I was worried about the shots. I was worried about the outcome. How did I handle it? As the pressure really mounted, I took a breather and reflected on just how far I had come. Yes, uncertainty lay ahead, but I had crossed a lot of stepping-stones to get to where I was standing. That gave me energy. That gave me courage.

I urge you to draw strength from all your experiences to date, and to prepare for your "big moment" by arming yourself with knowledge and facts. In this chapter you'll find information to help you understand how the IVF process works along with an up-close look at a typical cycle. In addition, I'll provide guidance on everything from choosing the best time for a cycle to keeping healthy—and calm!—during treatments. Well, we certainly have a lot of ground to cover so let's get started. Although no two IVF cycles are exactly alike, it's my hope that the pages that follow will offer the tools you need to enter into yours with optimism and confidence.

Understanding the Big Picture

Before we zoom in on what you'll need to know to gear up for your cycle, let's take a few minutes to pan across the entire process. After all, the better you understand the big picture, the better prepared you'll be for your treatments. Just ask Glenn. This 38-year-old product manager recalls: "I wanted a solid understanding of IVF so I could be there for my wife. But I have to admit I got off to a rocky start. The learning curve kind of reminded me of this course I took in college called 'Semiotics in Non-Western Society.' Like that class, I panicked first. There were so many new words to learn—*estradiol, gonadotropins, blastocyst*—that I got overwhelmed. And when I'm overwhelmed, I can't absorb new information. So I followed the strategy I used to survive Semiotics—I relaxed, set the vocabulary aside, and focused on the concept. After that, I calmed down and the process really clicked in!"

Glenn is right. Strip away in vitro's high-tech aura and intimidating jargon and you're left with a pretty straightforward process. And that process has a simple goal—to get you pregnant. Although the length of IVF cycles varies from patient to patient, most end up taking a little more than a month. Remember the six basics steps from Chapter 1? Let's look at them again:

Step 1: Suppression and Developing Eggs: During this two- to three-week phase, IVFers take Lupron (or an alternate drug, such as Antagon) to shut off normal ovulation. They then take one or more superovulatory medications to stimulate the maturation of multiple eggs.

Step 2: Retrieving Eggs: When the eggs are *almost* fully mature, an HCG shot is administered, which will release them from the ovaries about 40 hours later. REs carefully time egg retrievals to happen just *before* ovulation—or when the eggs are at the peak of their ripeness.

Step 3: Developing Embryos: After the eggs are collected, they're combined with sperm in lab dishes for fertilization. ICSI—the process of injecting a single sperm into an egg to jump-start fertilization—is used in about 50 percent of cases.

Step 4: Transferring Embryos: REs typically transfer two to four embryos into the uterus. If the couple has fewer high-quality embryos—say two to four—that transfer usually takes place three days after retrieval; if a couple has more healthy embryos—say five or more—the transfer usually takes place five days after retrieval.

Step 5: Preparing the Uterine Lining: Right around transfer time, women begin daily injections of progesterone to enrich the uterine lining and prepare it for incoming embryos. Progesterone supplements continue until the pregnancy test (and beyond if a pregnancy is achieved).

Step 6: Taking the Pregnancy Test: Although pregnancy test dates vary from practice to practice, most women take their first one about 10 days to 2 weeks after their transfer.

Kelli's IVF Calendar

Sunday	Monday	Tuesday	Wednesday
Day 1/ Cycle Begins • Period due in about 7 days • Start Lupron injections to turn off ovulation	**Day 2** • Lupron	**Day 3** • Lupron	**Day 4** • Lupron
Day 8 • Period arrives! Call IVF office to alert them • Lupron	**Day 9/ Stimulation Begins** • Office visit: Baseline blood test & ultrasound • Continue Lupron but reduce dosage • Start Superovulatory drugs to develop eggs	**Day 10** • Reduced Lupron • Superovulatory drugs	**Day 11** • Reduced Lupron • Superovulatory drugs
Day 15 • Office visit: Blood test & ultrasound to track eggs • Reduced Lupron • Reduced Superovulatory drugs	**Day 16** • Office visit: Blood test & ultrasound to track eggs • Reduced Lupron • Reduced Superovulatory drugs	**Day 17** • Office visit: Blood test & ultrasound to track eggs (Follicles are at 15 to 18 mm—GOAL!) • HCG shot at 12 AM!	**Day 18** • Antibiotic for both partners • Medrol
Day 22 • Progesterone • 7 embryos remain!	**Day 23** • Progesterone • 7 embryos remain!	**Day 24/ Transfer** • Office Visit: 2 embryos are transferred to the uterus (5 are frozen) • Bed rest for 24 hours • Progesterone	**Day 25** • Progesterone
Day 29 • Progesterone	**Day 30** • Progesterone	**Day 31** • Progesterone	**Day 32** • Progesterone

Thursday	Friday	Saturday
Day 5 • Lupron	**Day 6** • Lupron	**Day 7** • Lupron
Day 12 • Office visit: Blood test & ultrasound to track eggs • Reduced Lupron • Superovulatory drugs	**Day 13** • Reduced Lupron • Superovulatory drugs	**Day 14** • Office visit: Blood test & ultrasound to track eggs • Reduced Lupron • Reduced Superovulatory drugs (Eggs are growing quickly!)
Day 19/Retrieval • Office Visit: Eggs are retrieved at precisely 12 PM • Partner produces sperm sample • 12 eggs are retrieved and placed with sperm for fertilization!	**Day 20** • Begin progesterone injections to enrich the uterine lining • There are 9 early embryos!	**Day 21** • Progesterone • 8 embryos remain!
Day 26 • Progesterone	**Day 27** • Progesterone	**Day 28** • Progesterone
Day 33 • Progesterone	**Day 34/PG Test** • Office Visit: Pregnancy test • Nurse calls later that afternoon to tell patient she's in the very early stages of pregnancy! •Progesterone	**Day 35** • Progesterone

Now that wasn't so bad, was it? While no two protocols are exactly the same, each patient must move through every one of these steps to achieve a pregnancy. Have you got them down pat? (I didn't think so.) Because IVF terminology is rather tricky, I thought it would be helpful to take a close look at a sample cycle. On pages 172–173, you'll find a day-by-day calendar of a fictitious IVFer who we'll call Kelli. She's 34, has low FSH, and mild endometriosis. In other words, she's a good candidate for in vitro. Although Kelli—and her doting husband, Trent—are works of my imagination, her course of treatment is very real and, in fact, very typical. Take a few minutes to tour the calendar, then read the narrative that follows for a more detailed description of her experience.

Diary of a Standard Cycle

As the calendar reflects, Kelli underwent the standard IVF treatment plan dubbed the "long protocol." The long protocol is so named because it takes longer—approximately 30 to 35 days—than other leading protocols. (For information on them see page 191.) Although Kelli's cycle officially begins with the first shot of Lupron on day 1, daily doses of the birth control pill were taken for the prior month. While the birth control pill isn't right for every IVFer, this "precursor" to a cycle is fast becoming a key component in many women's protocols. Why? It grants REs a tighter rein on their patients' treatment by determining the start of menstruation, which usually determines the start of IVF. In addition, research suggests that it helps prevent ovarian cysts from forming and lays the groundwork for successful egg development.

Step 1: Suppression and Developing Eggs
Kelli's cycle—as for the majority of IVFers—kicks off with daily injections of a drug called Lupron, timed to begin one week prior to the arrival of her period. Lupron, a *gonadotropin-releasing hormone agonist,* has the important job of putting her ovaries to "sleep." Yes, it may sound counterintuitive to shut down ovulation when the goal of IVF

is to get you pregnant, but it actually makes sense. Why? Shutting down normal ovulation gives doctors the opportunity to control the course of a patient's cycle and reduces the risk of eggs being released from the ovaries before they can be retrieved. To administer the Lupron, our fictional protagonist Kelli pokes a half-inch needle into her thigh. This type of shot is known as a *subcutaneous injection* because it delivers the medication just under the skin. The very first shot is a bit nerve-racking, but she's pleasantly surprised when it barely registers a tingle. And there appear to be no major side effects except for an occasional headache. Both are a relief to her husband, Trent, who is a self-professed worrier.

For seven days straight, Kelli gives herself shots of Lupron and awaits her period. Kelli's doctor warned her to watch closely or she might miss it. He wasn't kidding! On day 8 of her IVF cycle, it comes. Between the birth control pill and the Lupron injections, her normal flow has been reduced to a few spots of brownish-red blood. That afternoon—as instructed—she phones her practice and reports that her period has arrived. A nurse then tells her to come into the office the following morning for tests.

On day 9 of her cycle (and the day after her period arrives), Kelli dutifully heads to her IVF clinic. There, a nurse draws blood to measure estradiol and her RE performs an ultrasound to confirm that her ovaries are quiet and that no cysts have formed. (Ovarian cysts, while not dangerous, can interfere with follicle growth and make monitoring the ovaries a challenge.) In late afternoon, Kelli receives a call from the nurse, who reports that all systems are go. The blood test and ultrasound confirmed that suppression is working. That means it's time to "awaken the eggs" and get them developing with superovulatory drugs. Kelli has been prescribed a combination of two—Gonal F and Repronex. The nurse tells her the exact dosages and instructs her to continue on Lupron, but to halve the amount (explaining that less is needed now that suppression has been achieved). That evening, Kelli injects the reduced Lupron and prepares the Gonal F and Repronex. Both are white powders that come packed in tiny glass bottles called *ampules*. Before her shots, Kelli has to mix the powders with a little saline water. The mixing business is rather intimidating, but she soon gets the hang of it. And as with the Lupron, she barely feels a thing. Let the egg maturation process begin!

For the next two evenings, day 10 and day 11, Kelli does exactly the same thing at the same hour: She gives herself an injection of reduced Lupron followed by injections of Gonal F and Repronex. The super-ovulatory drugs make her feel a bit moody and bloated, kind of like mild PMS. On the morning of day 12, Kelli returns to her IVF clinic for another blood test and ultrasound. Again, the nurse draws blood to measure her estradiol; a steady increase is a good sign. Again, the RE performs an ultrasound to check her ovaries; expanding follicles mean eggs are developing inside them. And there *are* expanding folli-cles—lots of them! In addition, the doctor takes a look at her uterine lining to make sure it's bulking up in preparation for incoming em-bryos. It is! (To help ensure successful implantation, doctors want to see a thickness of 9 millimeters or more.) Later that afternoon, as has become the custom, Kelli receives a call from the nurse. Things are progressing according to plan. She's told to continue her nightly ritual of reduced Lupron, Gonal F, and Repronex for the next few days.

As instructed, Kelli takes her medications; each day, she feels a little moodier, a little more bloated. There's even an occasional hot flash. Although side effects vary from patient to patient, it's pretty typical for them to become more severe as treatment ramps up. On day 14, Kelli ventures to her IVF clinic for another blood test and ultrasound. The doctor reports that her egg-filled follicles appear to be growing nicely. He points out a scattering of tiny dark dots on the ultrasound screen— these are the developing follicles. He then counts and measures them. Later that afternoon, Kelli receives a call from the nurse. Things are going well, but her follicles are growing a little faster than planned and the RE wants to slow them down by reducing her dosage of Gonal F and Repronex. Adjusting the dosage of her superovulatory drugs is rather like easing up—or bearing down—on the gas pedal of a car to help patients arrive at the egg retrieval stage at just the right time.

On days 15, 16, and 17, Kelli makes the morning pilgrimage to her IVF office. Now that the egg-maturing portion of her cycle is in full swing, her RE wants to see her every day. On days 15 and 16, she's told to continue the same dosage of Lupron and superovulatory drugs, but on day 17 the nurse calls with some exciting news: Her blood test and ultrasound indicate that her eggs are approaching their goal. Fully mature follicles measure 18 to 23 millimeters in diameter and some of Kelli's are in that range. Plus Kelli's uterine lining is bulking up perfectly—measuring more than 9 millimeters in thickness. That means egg retrieval is just around the corner!

The nurse tells Kelli to discontinue the Lupron and superovulatory drugs. Instead, at midnight on the dot, her husband is to give her an injection of *human chorionic gonadotropin* (HCG). The nurse explains that this special shot is like pushing a button to trigger ovulation in roughly 40 hours. However, ovulation won't happen. Why? Kelli's RE plans to collect the ripe-and-ready eggs a few hours before that deadline.

Because the HCG must be delivered to muscle tissue, it gets injected into Kelli's upper butt cheek via an inch-and-a-half-long needle. This type of shot is known as an *intramuscular injection*. That means Trent will have to do the honors. The needle's a little scary-looking, but he manages the task just fine. The shot does sting a bit, but it also marks the halfway point of Kelli's cycle.

Step 2: Retrieving Eggs

Day 18—the morning after Kelli's HCG shot—feels like the calm before the storm. The button has been pushed for ovulation the following day. In the meantime, there's little to do. The Lupron and superovulatory injections are over. In fact, her only two tasks are to take Medrol, an oral steroid to aid implantation, along with an antibiotic to prevent the slim chance of infection during the forthcoming egg retrieval. Trent has to take an antibiotic, too. For him, the purpose is to help reduce the amount of bacteria in his sperm. Bacteria could compromise the sperm's performance during fertilization. (Because Kelli will be undergoing anesthesia during egg retrieval, she's instructed not to eat or drink anything after midnight.)

On day 19, Kelli and Trent excitedly head over to their IVF clinic—careful not to be late. Because the retrieval is precisely timed to enable the collection of eggs just before ovulation, it's essential that they're punctual. At noon, Kelli dons a hospital gown and lies down on a table. An IV containing a sedative is connected to her arm and before she can say *10, 9, 8* . . . she's out. As she sleeps, a special syringe is inserted through her vagina and it reaches to her ovaries. Then, guided by ultrasound images, her RE gently sucks the mature eggs out of their follicles. A mere twenty minutes later, Kelli is awakened. She feels a bit groggy, but there's no pain.

As Kelli rests comfortably, Trent's off on assignment. In a quiet room, he's masturbating to generate the sperm that will be used to fertilize her eggs. The pressure is on! Still, with the aid of a few steamy magazines he gets the job done. (During a previous visit, he has produced backup sperm that has been prefrozen just in case.) When he's through, the couple is reunited and gets some encouraging news: 12 healthy eggs were retrieved!

Step 3: Developing Embryos

As the couple heads home to take it easy, the embryologist—or doctor in charge of the fertilization process—has much to do. First, Trent's sperm are washed, spun, and tested. Next, 50,000 to 100,000 of the healthiest specimens are placed in each of the twelve nutrient-rich lab dishes containing Kelli's eggs. Talk about survival of the fittest! A given egg will be fertilized by only a single sperm.

On day 20, the doctor uses a high-powered microscope to peer into each dish. Eureka! He sees the first tentative signs of fertilization: the formation of two clear bubbles on the egg called *the pronuclei*. One represents the genetic contribution of the male and the other represents the genetic contribution of the female. Later that day, nine of Kelli's eggs have converted to very early embryos. Most of these embryos continue to develop, but a few don't make it. Embryos with chromosomal defects tend to peter out rather than divide. By day 21, eight remain, and by day 22, there are only seven. Their RE assures the couple that losing embryos along the way is perfectly normal, and he has some encouraging news: The remaining seven look healthy and strong. In fact, he gives each one the coveted grade of "excellent."

Step 4: Transferring Embryos

Most patients have their eggs transferred to the uterus three days after retrieval, but sometimes REs wait a full five days to do the job.

The reason? When a couple has a large number of high-quality embryos, it makes sense to allow them to divide and redivide in the lab dishes, then pick the heartiest ones to transfer. Which are deemed the heartiest? Quickly dividing embryos with even, symmetrical cells. Embryos transferred three days after retrieval usually have four to eight cells, but embryos transferred five days after retrieval sometimes have as many as 100 cells! While both types of transfers are very effective, those completed at the five-day "blastocyst" stage stand the very best chance of surviving in utero.

As their embryos develop in the lab dishes, Kelli and Trent are given periodic progress reports. When it's clear that seven are thriving, doctors opt for a five-day "blastocyst" transfer. On day 24, Kelli and Trent arrive at their IVF practice, giddy with anticipation. Today is transfer day! Since the couple is relatively young and their embryos are rated "excellent," it's decided that only two will be transferred. That way, if all goes well, Kelli will become pregnant with a singleton or twins—but not triplets (which could pose health risks to her and her babies). It's also decided that the remaining embryos will be frozen for possible use in future cycles.

During the transfer, Kelli lies on a table with her feet in stirrups. Trent holds her hand. He also clutches two blurry photos of cell masses magnified multiple times. (It is not uncommon for practices to give IVFers microscope pictures of the embryos to be transferred to help them with visualization.) *Will these be the first photos in our baby album?* he wonders. Next, the RE places a special catheter through Kelli's cervical canal, then gently injects both embryos into her uterus. The whole process takes a couple minutes and is utterly painless. Perhaps too painless? Kelli feels nothing, which alarms her a bit. After all, shouldn't she feel *something* during this momentous occasion? Her RE assures her that feeling nothing is perfectly normal. Even that hypersensitive fairy-tale princess—the one who feels a pea beneath 100 mattresses—could not detect the presence of such tiny embryos. Her doctor explains that they will drift around in her uterus for a few days and then, provided all goes well, attach to her uterine wall. Kelli rests for half an hour before being discharged. Even though there is no hard evidence to suggest that bed rest aids implantation, her doctor errs on the side of caution by asking her to lie down for the next 24 hours.

Step 5: Preparing the Uterus

Although the transfer occurs on day 24, the prepping of the uterine lining begins a few days earlier. As you can see from the calendar, Kelli starts daily injections of progesterone on day 20. Why? Progesterone—a naturally occurring hormone—enriches the uterine lining, creating the optimal conditions for embryos to stick and stay. Like the HCG shot, progesterone is injected into her upper butt cheek. Of all the shots, these are the toughest. Because the progesterone is thick and oily, it takes a while for the viscous fluid to exit the needle and enter her muscle. Even so, the momentary throbbing isn't too bad.

Step 6: Taking the Pregnancy Test(s)

On day 26, two days after her transfer, Kelli returns to work filled with hope and fear. Hope, because there's a good chance she's pregnant; fear, because there's also a good chance she's not. The odds of a good candidate like Kelli achieving pregnancy are about 50–50. During this nine-day waiting period, she listens intently to her body. On day 28, she's "sure" that she's pregnant; on day 30, she's "sure" that she's not. The truth is, at this early stage and with so much progesterone in her system, it's impossible to know anything for certain. Kelli finds this phase of the cycle the hardest—following weeks of treatment, there is nothing to do but wait.

Finally, on day 34, she and Trent pay a nerve-jangled visit to the IVF clinic for a very early pregnancy test. One simple prick and they're sent home to await the results. While they count the minutes, Kelli's blood is being tested for HCG—a hormone produced by an implanted embryo. If its detected, it will be a promising sign.

For several hours, they train their attention on the telephone. When it finally rings, Kelli's heart is in her throat. She answers and the nurse asks if she's sitting down. Kelli lowers herself into a chair, clutching Trent's hand. "It's too early to tell for sure," reports the nurse, "but your HCG level is pretty elevated, which may mean that you're pregnant with twins!" Kelli leaps to her feet; Trent does his signature happy jig. Formal congratulations would be premature: The couple won't have a definitive read on the status of her pregnancy until a fetal heartbeat—or two—is detected in about six weeks. Still, the signs are auspicious. And there is ample reason for Kelli and Trent to be hopeful that their dream of parenthood will soon become a reality.

How REs Customize IVF Protocols

As you read this, thousands of women are embarking upon IVF cycles all across the country. While many of them will be following a protocol quite similar to Kelli's, others will be undergoing variations, which include small or sizable tweaks to medications and timetables. In a way, designing a treatment plan is a bit like fitting a woman for shoes. Sure, the majority of us wear a size seven or eight, but plenty will need a size five or six or ten-and-a-half. When it comes to in vitro, one size most certainly does not fit all! The best REs know this and work hard to create appropriate protocols for every patient they serve. How do they make their decisions? First and foremost, they take into account the woman's:

- fertility issue(s)

- age

- Day-Three FSH level

- outstanding health concerns

- partner's sperm quality

- previous IVF cycles (if any)

A 41-year-old with elevated FSH, for example, will likely require a larger dose of superovulatory meds than a 30-year-old with a blocked tube. "It's not uncommon for patients we believe to be 'poor responders' to receive two or even four times the amount of stimulation drugs as some others," reports Dr. Daniel Stein, head of the IVF program at St. Luke's Hospital in New York City. Why is this the case? Women with diminished ovarian reserves tend to need more "fertilizer" to effectively mature the eggs that remain. Then, there are those IVFers who respond *too well* to superovulatory meds. A twentysomething in the prime of her fertility or someone with polycystic ovaries, for example, runs the risk of becoming overstimulated, which can lead to the formation of ovarian cysts or even a rare but dangerous condition known as ovarian hyperstimulation syndrome (OHSS). (For more information on the latter see pages 203 and 229.) To avoid these pitfalls, REs meticulously monitor each patient's estrogen level (through blood tests) and follicle growth (through ultrasounds). If follicles are growing too quickly, they ease up on the gas pedal by reducing the dose of superovulatory drugs; conversely, if follicles are growing too slowly, they accelerate growth by upping the dose.

Another important tool REs have at their disposal is their trusty menu of superovulatory medications—each a little different from the next. (See page 185 for a list.) Back in the early days of in vitro, the only type available were *human menopausal gonadotropins,* a family of meds derived from the urine of postmenopausal women. That's right, postmenopausal woman. You see, older women produce and excrete excess follicle-stimulating hormone (FSH) and luteinizing hormone (LH)—two hormones that stimulate follicles to grow. I know it sounds a little icky, but rest assured the urine is distilled, purified, and perfectly safe. And the regimen was—and is—pretty darn effective: Hundreds of thousands of IVFers have achieved healthy pregnancies with these gonadotropins. Common brands include Repronex and Bravelle. Still, they don't work for everyone.

Enter genetically engineered superovulatory drugs. In the early 1990s, advancements in science made it possible to produce a new breed of follicle-growing medication by placing synthetic genes in Chinese hamster ovaries, then manipulating them in a lab to make FSH. You heard right, *hamster* ovaries. Thanks to this technology, two highly effective medications were added to the IVF menu—Gonal F and Follistim. Today, they're the most popular choice for in vitro. Their edge over urinary gonadotropins? They don't contain as many impurities, are more consistent from batch to batch, and, perhaps most importantly, are devoid of LH. Although a little LH is necessary to mature eggs, all women produce it naturally to varying degrees and too much can inhibit the maturation of healthy eggs. For that reason, this new type of lab-generated medication is just what the doctor ordered for many IVFers, especially those with polycystic ovary disease.

Just as most folks have their favorite ice cream flavors, most REs have their favorite superovulatory drugs and drug combinations. Some patients take one and some take two. Perhaps the most common scenario is for women to take a genetically engineered drug *along with* a smaller dose of a human menopausal gonadotropin. That enables REs to add a little LH to the mix, but not too much. During my second IVF cycle, for example, I was given Gonal F plus Repronex. Why? Because that's the duo that my doctor found usually worked best for others like me. Different types of patients thrive on different types of drugs. Seasoned REs are acutely aware of this and carefully fine-tune each prescription to address each IVFer's individual needs.

Another medication that REs fine-tune is Lupron. Remember that all-important drug that turns off ovulation? The correct dosage is key. Why? A surplus can sometimes cause too much suppression, making it hard for the superovulatory drugs to wake up a woman's eggs and get them maturing. Thus, some IVFers—especially those who are older—are given smaller doses for shorter spans of time. In addition, a few are given Antagon or Centrotide instead. These two new drugs have only been available in the United States since 2000. But many REs are finding that these "suppression substitutes" work better than Lupron for certain patients, especially those with diminished ovarian reserves. They also have the benefit of working much quicker than Lupron, often requiring only a couple of days of injections.

What other variables do REs have to add to the mix? The birth control pill, for one. Prescribing the pill to IVFers a month prior to their cycle seems to help set the stage for quality eggs and reduce the likelihood of ovarian cysts forming. Doctors also choose from a menu of diverse medications to aid implantation, including estrogen, aspirin, heparin, nitroglycerin patches, even Viagra. Yup, Viagra is not just for men these days! Studies suggest that it increases the blood supply to the uterus, which helps some women with too-thin linings bulk them up. In addition, doctors rely on a bag of microscopic tricks to foster fertilization, including ICSI, the injection of a single sperm directly into an egg, and assisted hatching, in which a teeny hole is drilled into an embryo to help it "hatch out" and implant in the uterine wall. Last but not least, REs carefully evaluate every developing embryo and make careful decisions about which ones are the very best candidates for transfer.

Fertility Fact: Gonal F and Follistim, the two most popular superovulatory drugs used in IVF, are created by genetically engineering the cells of hamster ovaries.

OK, I think you get the drift. Although a portfolio of basic treatment plans exists (see Five Important IVF Protocols on page 191), seldom are two cycles exactly alike. That's a good thing. The best REs customize each woman's protocol based on research, observation, and previous experience treating similar patients. Also, they're willing to pick up the phone when they're uncertain about how to proceed. "If I'm not sure about the best way to treat someone," reports Dr. Daniel Stein, "I'll call an RE that I respect and say, 'What would you do with this type of patient?'"

Is there a superior protocol out there? Quite simply, no. It's important to understand that different treatment plans work for different patients. Do REs have all the answers all the time? Unfortunately not. Infertility science is still a relatively new discipline and, frankly, plenty of mystery remains. Sometimes in-vitro candidates come along and—try as they might—REs can't come up with the right "recipe" to get them pregnant. That being said, the general hit rate is pretty impressive and getting better every day. Experts estimate that about 70 percent of today's IVFers achieve their goal of parenthood within one to three tries.

Medication Menu

The following is a menu of the most popular drugs used for IVF today. (Not to worry, you'll only need a few of these.) Your RE will work carefully to pick and choose the very best combination to maximize your chances of achieving a pregnancy. Self-medicating can throw a wrench into even the most promising cycles so be sure not to take anything—not even aspirin!—without speaking to your doctor first.

Medication Menu

To Set the Stage for High-Quality Eggs: Since the late 1990s, REs have been adding the birth control pill to the protocols of many IVFers.

- **The Birth Control Pill:** Many patients take the birth control pill for one to several weeks prior to the start of their cycle to help REs synchronize treatment plans and reduce the occurrence of ovarian cysts. Women with blood-clotting disorders should not take it.

  Delivery: oral

  Possible Side Effects: bloating, changes in appetite, nausea, headaches, breast tenderness, moodiness

- -

To "Turn Off" Normal Ovulation: REs choose one of these medications to suppress ovulation.

- **Lupron:** Since the late 1980s, this synthetic hormone has been a staple of most IVF cycles. The bottle should be refrigerated after the first use.

  Delivery: subcutaneous injection

Medication Menu *(continued on next page)*

Medication Menu *(continued)*

Possible Side Effects: headaches, hot flashes, sweats, breast tenderness, constipation, dizziness, fatigue, moodiness, vaginal dryness, irritation at injection site

- **Synarel:** Like Lupron, this drug shuts down ovulation. Although popular in Europe, stateside IVF programs seldom use it because it is considered slightly less effective.

   Delivery: nasal spray

   Possible Side Effects: headaches, hot flashes, sweats, breast tenderness, constipation, dizziness, fatigue, moodiness, vaginal dryness, nose irritation

- **Antagon, Centrotide:** Certified by the FDA in 2000, these promising new suppression drugs appear to be a good option for many IVFers—especially "poor responders." Because they work more quickly than Lupron, most IVFers need only take Antagon or Centrotide for four days or less. In fact, some patients require only a single shot of Centrotide to achieve effective suppression!

   Delivery: subcutaneous injection

   Possible Side Effects: abdominal pain and/or swelling, nausea, diarrhea, weight gain, irritation at injection site

----

To Stimulate Egg Development: REs usually prescribe one or a combination of two of these superovulatory drugs to foster the ripening of multiple eggs.

- **Repronex:** This superovulatory drug contains natural hormones derived from the urine of postmenopausal women. It's made up of 50 percent follicle stimulating hormone and 50 percent luteinizing hormone.

   Delivery: subcutaneous injection

Medication Menu *(continued)*

Possible Side Effects: bloating, fluid retention, breast tenderness, nausea, moodiness, fatigue, restlessness

- **Bravelle:** This medication is also derived from the urine of postmenopausal women, but is highly purified to remove most of the luteinizing hormone. As a result, it contains mostly follicle stimulating hormone with just a hint of luteinizing hormone.

  Delivery: subcutaneous injection

  Possible Side Effects: bloating, fluid retention, breast tenderness, nausea, moodiness, fatigue, restlessness

- **Follistim, Gonal F:** These two popular brands are very similar. Both are genetically engineered in a lab, and so they contain fewer impurities and are more consistent from batch to batch than those derived from postmenopausal urine. These medications contain follicle stimulating hormone, but no luteinizing hormone.

  Delivery: subcutaneous injection

  Possible Side Effects: bloating, fluid retention, breast tenderness, nausea, moodiness, fatigue, restlessness

---

To Prepare Ripe Eggs for Retrieval: The human chorionic gonadotropin (HCG) injection is ordered when eggs are closing in on their peak of maturity. Expect egg retrieval about 36 hours after the shot.

- **Navarel, Pregnyl, Profasi:** Like the majority of the superovulatory drugs listed above, these brands of HCG come from human urine—but this time it's that of pregnant women. This hormone, produced by the placenta, triggers the release of eggs from the ovaries roughly 40 hours after the injection is administered.

Medication Menu *(continued on next page)*

Medication Menu *(continued)*

Delivery: intramuscular injection

Possible Side Effects: bloating, breast enlargement, headaches, nausea, constipation, irritation at injection site

• **Ovidrel:** This new, genetically engineered form of HCG contains few impurities and can be administered with the "short" needle. Expect it to gain popularity in years to come.

Delivery: subcutaneous injection

Possible Side Effects: bloating, breast enlargement, headaches, nausea, constipation, irritation at injection site

---

To Foster a Successful Egg Retrieval: During this important step, both partners benefit from a few familiar medications.

• **Doxycycline, Tetracycline:** Around egg-retrieval time, women take an antibiotic to reduce the already slim chance of infection. Men, too, are sometimes prescribed an antibiotic to help ensure a healthy, bacteria-free sperm sample.

Delivery: oral

Possible Side Effects: restlessness, sensitivity to sunlight, gastrointestinal distress, yeast infections (in women)

• **Medrol:** This steroid mildly suppresses the immune system to decrease the chances of the body rejecting incoming embryos.

Delivery: oral

Possible Side Effects: rashes, nausea, headaches, low blood pressure (rare)

To Promote Implantation: Although progesterone is the single most important medication to promote healthy implantation, REs sometimes augment it with other drugs on a case-by-case basis.

- **Progesterone:** This naturally occurring hormone enriches the uterine lining to help embryos stick and stay put. Most IVFers are prescribed injectable progesterone in oil, but the use of suppositories or vaginal gels (such as Crinone) are becoming more widespread.

    Delivery: intramuscular injection, suppositories, or vaginal gel

    Possible Side Effects: cramping, constipation, diarrhea, nausea, headaches, breast tenderness, joint pain, drowsiness, nervousness, increased urination at night

- **Baby Aspirin:** Taken daily, a single low-dose aspirin seems to keep placental blood vessels open to aid implantation.

    Delivery: oral

    Possible Side Effects: allergic reaction, nausea (both rare)

- **Heparin:** This blood thinner is often prescribed to women with antiphospholipid antibodies to increase blood flow to their uterus and thwart clotting, which can trigger early miscarriage.

    Delivery: subcutaneous injection

    Possible Side Effects: chills, fever, headache, nausea, vomiting, rashes, irritation at injection site

- **Estrace:** To help progesterone prepare the uterine lining, some patients receive this synthetic estrogen supplement as well. It's also a

Medication Menu *(continued on next page)*

Medication Menu *(continued)*

standard ingredient in the protocols for women undergoing frozen cycles or donor-egg cycles, or acting as gestational surrogates.

Delivery: oral

Possible Side Effects: bloating, nausea, breast tenderness, and, in extreme cases: leg numbness, chest pains, visual disturbances, shortness of breath (the latter symptoms should be reported to your RE immediately)

• **Viagra:** A few REs prescribe Viagra to help women with especially thin uterine lining bulk them up. How does it work? The drug appears to increase blood flow to the uterus and in so doing thickens the walls.

Delivery: vaginal suppositories

Possible Side Effects: none reported

To Help Ensure a Healthy Pregnancy: Like all women hoping to conceive, IVFers are encouraged to take daily doses of folic acid and a multivitamin a few months before treatment to set the stage for a successful pregnancy and reduce the chance of birth defects.

• **Multivitamin:** A vitamin a day helps ensure that both mother and baby-to-be receive essential nutrients.

Delivery: oral

Possible Side Effects: constipation, nausea

• **Folic Acid:** Research shows that folic acid taken in the early stages of pregnancy—and just before!—helps prevent birth defects.

Delivery: oral

Possible Side Effects: fever, rashes, itching (rare)

Five Important IVF Protocols

Here's a list of some notable treatment plans that are commonly performed in the United States:

- **Long Protocol:** Some variation of this popular treatment plan—also referred to as "Lupron Down-Regulation"—is used in at least half of all U.S. cycles. Outlined earlier in Diary of a Standard Cycle, it's the protocol of choice for those considered strong candidates for IVF.

- **Flare Protocol:** In women with poor ovarian reserves, Lupron can sometimes cause too much suppression, which inhibits egg development once the stimulation phase of IVF kicks in. This protocol addresses the problem by starting Lupron just a day prior to superovulatory drugs. That way, women take a lot less Lupron. In addition, this timetable enables doctors to take advantage of the surge—or "flare"—of FSH and LH that occurs when Lupron is first given to "fire up" follicle growth.

- **Micro-Flare Protocol:** This aggressive therapy is sometimes the treatment of choice for women with a poor IVF prognosis because of advanced age or poor egg quality. It's similar to the Flare Protocol except *even less* Lupron is given to avoid oversuppression. Although the success rates aren't nearly as high as with the Long Protocol, it sometimes manages to do the trick.

- **Antagonist Protocol:** In 2000, the Federal Drug Administration certified *antagonist*—brand names Antagon and Centrotide—for use in the United States. Because it's new on the scene, there is still much to learn about this medication that turns off ovulation. Although the jury is still out, a number of REs are big fans. Using it in place of Lupron appears to work well for certain candidates, especially older ones. Plus, IVFers need only take it for four or fewer days.

- **Natural-Cycle Protocol:** Although not widely available, the natural-cycle protocol is the perfect option for the rare IVFer who's either resistant to or intolerant to fertility medications. In this treatment, no drugs are used. Instead the patient is closely monitored during her natural ovulation cycle and a single egg is retrieved, fertilized, and transferred at the blastocyst stage. The disadvantage is that success rates are far lower than with standard cycles. The advantage, however, is that it's far less costly and requires no medication.

Getting Set to Cycle

I hope that you found the sample cycle and information on how REs design protocols helpful. Still have some lingering questions regarding certain aspects of the process? Not to worry. I'll zoom in on the specifics of what to expect during your own IVF cycle in the next chapter. In the meantime, I wanted to give you the heads-up on a few more orders of business that will need to be taken care of before embarking on treatment. The green light to do in vitro is a graduation of sorts. It means a good part of your journey—namely, finding out what's wrong and locating a good practice—is now behind you. It also indicates that you've "passed" a number of prerequisite exams, including the all-important Day-Three FSH Test, an evaluation of your ovaries and uterus, a bunch of cervical cultures, and a batch of obligatory blood tests to rule out everything from hepatitis C to German measles. (For a complete list of necessary tests, see page 129.)

In addition, REs usually perform a "mock transfer." Fear not, this procedure sounds like a bigger deal than it actually is. During this simple test, which usually takes place some time before the start of a cycle, a small plastic catheter is inserted into the patient's vagina. This enables REs to measure the depth and direction of her uterus. That way, there'll be no surprises at actual transfer time and doctors will have a road map of sorts to help them guide the embryos to their important destination. April, a 33-year-old production editor, recalls, "I was kind of nervous about the mock transfer, but it only took about five minutes. There was a little cramping and that was it."

Many practices also do an antral follicle count. During this test, usually conducted at the start of menstruation, REs take a close look at a patient's ovaries via ultrasound. Then, they count the number of *antral follicles*—small, developing, egg-containing follicles—they see. A high number of visible antral follicles (say 20 to 30) is a strong indicator that the patient will produce numerous eggs during IVF. By the same token, a low count (under 7) indicates that she will not. While no test is 100 percent accurate, some doctors consider the antral follicle count among their best tools to predict outcomes and plan medication dosages. They know, for example, that women with many antral follicles will likely require a lower dose of superovulatory drugs to stimulate follicle growth than women with few.

No question, requisite pokes and prods aren't a picnic, but they are a rite of passage. They help doctors plan the best course of treatment for your individual needs. Another rite of passage is getting a general sense of your chances of succeeding with in vitro fertilization.

Understanding Your Chances for Success

Getting the go-ahead for a cycle is a vote of confidence that you're a good candidate for in vitro. In the context of IVF, however, "good candidate" has a pretty broad definition. It can mean anything from your doctor believes you're a shoo-in to get pregnant, to your doctor believes there's a slim chance he or she can help you to achieve your goal. Ethical REs won't take on patients with extremely poor prognoses for standard cycles. (Instead, they point them toward egg donation or adoption.) But many of them *will* take on challenging cases, in which the odds for success are far less than 50–50. Why? They believe they owe it to these patients to try to help them. Likewise, some of the patients believe they owe it to themselves to explore the IVF option before ruling it out.

Fertility Fact: A recent study found that IVF cycles begun in spring result in minutely higher birth rates than those begun in winter.

What are your ballpark chances of success? To find out, it's a good idea to have a heart-to-heart with your RE *before* committing to a cycle. This can happen in person or over the phone, but it should be at a time when your doctor can provide undivided attention. "We work hard to educate patients about their success rates," remarks Dr. Brad Kolb, a seasoned RE at Huntington Reproductive Center in Pasadena, California. How do doctors like Kolb make their assessments? They carefully consider a candidate's age, fertility factors, and test results, then mentally crunch the numbers. Because every IVFer is unique, it goes without saying that it's impossible to provide "real" success rates. Still, a good RE should be able to make a well-founded conjecture. Some will quote a statistical rate and others will rely on a telling adjective such as *excellent, very good, so-so,* and *poor.* If possible, draw your doctor out and ask him or her to explain the thinking behind the assessment.

Knowing where you stand can feel a bit like staring directly into the sun. Even so, it's essential information. Optimism is a great tool for everyone, but there's benefit to knowing the facts. Walking around with blinders on may help you sail through a cycle, but it won't do you much good if that cycle fails. Everyone should hope for the best—for there is much reason to be hopeful!—but they should also prepare for the possibility of failure. Even "excellent" candidates with all the right bells and whistles don't always get pregnant. Just as women with several seeming strikes against them sometimes do. Bethany, a 41-year-old architect, recalls her IVF efforts: "My doctor was pretty honest: I was a C minus candidate at best. But she thought it was definitely worth trying. Armed with that information, my husband and I decided to move forward with a cycle or two. Our thinking was that we didn't want to look back on this opportunity and not take it. If it failed, yes, we'd be sad but at least we would have tried. Well, all I can say is, I'm glad we went for it. We were lucky, really, really lucky: I got pregnant after my first attempt!"

Fact: A percentage of women who look like poor candidates on paper manage to achieve healthy pregnancies with IVF. And those whose first cycle ends in a negative pregnancy test, as mine did, should bear in mind that in vitro is a process, not a single-shot attempt at pregnancy. One failure doesn't mean that it won't work down the road, especially in cases where REs reflect upon and amend patient protocols. I realize it's not easy to hear that success may require additional tries—not to mention additional cash—but it's wise to have a flexible game plan in place for pursuing future cycles if your first one doesn't work. Quitting after a single try is certainly the right choice for some, but not all. For me, it would have been like opting out of the marathon I'd trained hard for at the halfway mark. No question IVF was a challenge—both mentally and physically—but, like Bethany, I'm really glad I kept on going.

Quick Tips for Dealing with Doctors and Nurses

OK, now that I've hammered home the importance of getting a ball-park assessment of your chances of success, I wanted to make you aware of another issue: Most REs are very, very busy. On any given day, they might be juggling a dozen or more patients and protocols, not to mention retrievals, transfers, mountains of paperwork, and, quite possibly, a teaching post and/or a research study. Doctors are important and dedicated people, but *so* are you. Don't lose sight of that fact. You're probably spending thousands of dollars on treatment and you clearly have a lot at stake. That means you deserve your RE's time and focus, regardless of his or her workload. "Knowledge is key. All patients can and should ask their doctors a lot of questions," stresses Dr. Jane Frederick, a respected RE at Huntington Reproductive Center in Pasadena, California.

There you have it, straight from an IVF doctor. Still, it's wise to be realistic—and canny—about getting your needs met. With all the stress of a cycle, the last thing you need is to start resenting your doctor because of perceived slights. Raquel, a 40-year-old stock analyst, shared her story with me: "Admittedly, I'm a strong personality. I'm accustomed to getting what I want, when I want it. So when my doctor took a long time to return my calls, it made me angry, which made me tense. 'This is not good,' I said to myself. To defuse the situation, I asked him how we could remedy the situation. After a little back and forth, we made a deal: I would leave my questions with his assistant, who would jot them down verbatim. Then he would call me back with answers in the evening, leaving detailed messages on my machine if I was unavailable."

Raquel's strategy was smart. Instead of getting frustrated, she focused on her end game—getting answers—and crafted a plan to effectively communicate with her busy doctor. I urge you to do the same. At the outset of treatments, have a conversation with your RE about receiving timely responses to your queries. Getting your doctor on the phone the second you punch in the digits is probably a pipe dream, but getting a call back by the end of the day is totally realistic. In addition, ask your RE about the possibility of corresponding via e-mail. Amanda, a 42-year-old homemaker, recalls: "When I had a question, I dashed off an e-mail to my doctor. Her responses were brief—some arriving in the wee small hours. But getting everything in writing was a definite plus." Is e-mail an option for you? You won't know unless you ask. The important thing is to have access to the information you need and deserve. That being said, the expertise of an RE isn't always required. As mentioned in a previous chapter, it makes sense to sort your IVF-related queries into separate piles for your RE, his or her assistant, a billing clerk, and a nurse. Here are a few examples:

- A question about your protocol—RE

- A question about scheduling your cycle—RE's assistant

- A question about paying—billing clerk

- A question about mixing medication—nurse

Assistants, billing clerks, and especially nurses are fantastic resources. Many, in fact, are *better* equipped than docs to field your questions—and usually far more available. My advice? Make it a point to get to know some key staff members at your IVF center. If someone is particularly accommodating in the billing department, for example, take the time to pay that person a well-deserved compliment. Then, ask if you can call on him or her directly in the future. Chances are that employees will be eager to maintain a reputation as efficient and helpful. It's a win-win situation: They feel good; you feel good!

This tip can and should be extended to nurses. Instead of playing the field, try to forge a partnership with a single nurse. Many of the nurses affiliated with IVF are amazingly kind and caring. They're also fonts of information—many having been intimately involved in hundreds of previous cycles. Got a question about giving shots? Super-ovulatory side effects? Early signs of pregnancy? A good nurse will have the answers to all these inquiries and more, usually without the intimidating doctor-speak. When I did IVF, a friend suggested that I cozy up to a nurse to act as my unofficial advocate. Yes, the campaign felt a little rehearsed, but I did it anyway. I struck up a rapport with a red-haired nurse with a nurturing manner and a wise smile. Looks didn't deceive. She was warm, dedicated, and supersmart. When I asked if I could contact her with questions, she was touched. And, I might add, she was meticulous about returning every phone call as promptly as possible.

Many women I interviewed for this book took the same approach. According to Sally, a 27-year-old actuary: "My doctor was great, but businesslike and very busy so I started calling a nurse named Marinka with most of my concerns. One day I freaked out about doing a shot, and she talked me down and saved the cycle. She was there every step of the way and even called me with my pregnancy results. I got pregnant and she got red roses!"

Choosing the Optimum Time for Treatments

Once you've passed the IVF audition, your doctor may be eager to slot you in to start your cycle immediately. In the name of efficiency, many in-vitro centers like to keep a steady flow of patients moving through the process. While scheduling you right away may make life easier for them, it may not be easier for you. Why? IVF is a four- to five-week commitment that requires a great deal of focus. Hastily shoehorning it into a time frame loaded with work obligations, travel, or important social events can add to your stress—and even affect your outcome. Nonetheless, you don't want to lose precious momentum by waiting too long. Plus, for those over 37, every month that passes subtly reduces fertility. Will a couple months make a difference? Probably not. But a couple years may.

So how do you decide on an optimal timetable? Tip number one: Know thy period. In vitro start dates are based on your menstrual cycle. As the possibility of treatment draws near, it's smart to have a log of last month's menstrual cycle at your fingertips. That way, when the nurse asks you to provide it, you won't get flustered or have to do the calculations in your head. Tip number two: Be aware that most IVF centers shut down for a few weeks during the winter holidays as well as in the summer to regroup. Make sure to have these dates handy, so your best-laid plans don't conflict with their downtime.

Tip number three: When your in-vitro clinic suggests a date, pencil it in, and ask to sleep on it. Then, go home and mull over the tentative schedule with your mate. After all, he'll be acting as your coach and should be available to support you through as much of the process as possible. Are the decks clear for both of you? Think hard. Did a monster sales meeting slip your mind? How about a business trip to Singapore, or Baltimore, or the fact that you've promised to play bridesmaid at a relative's wedding? (It's surprising how easily key commitments can get jumbled.) "I made a mistake," laughs Penelope, a 33-year-old pharmaceutical rep. "I scheduled my IVF cycle smack-dab in the middle of a close cousin's wedding. I ended up hiking my bridesmaid dress in the bathroom to get my shot while the Macarena blared in the background. I got through it, but all the wedding obligations made it far more challenging than it had to be."

Sure, there are probably a few type A (plus!) women reading this book who actually relish the adrenaline-jacked challenge of balancing work and travel, social obligations and treatments. More power to you. But for the rest, why play superwoman when you don't have to? If the next two months look particularly hellish, simply wait until your calendar opens up to begin your cycle. Or, consider doing in vitro during your allotted vacation time. Sure, going across town to the clinic for tests every day isn't as exotic as snorkeling in the tropics, but it might reduce your stress level—and save you a few bucks in the process. "I'm a first-grade teacher," reports 28-year-old Jeri. "I have to be at work at 7:30 A.M. sharp. That made treatments during the school year totally impossible. How did I spend my summer vacation? Seeing movies, going to museums—and doing IVF. It was a great solution. Plus the money I saved by *not* going away went straight into my treatment fund."

Like Jeri, it's wise to plan carefully and pick a chunk of time that's wide open so you can train all your attention on your goal—getting pregnant. But don't postpone the decision for too long. Select an appropriate start date, then call your IVF practice and ask them to put you on the official schedule. If you drag your feet, their calendar may fill up with other candidates. And the last thing you want is to get bumped because there are no remaining spots open. Believe me, it happens.

Balancing Work and Treatments

Remember my friend Lucy from Chapter 5? During her IVF treatments, she schlepped—as we New Yorkers like to say—all the way from Brooklyn to Stamford, Connecticut. That's where the sole practice that actually accepted her insurance was located. How the heck did she manage? By prying her eyes open at 4:45 A.M., hopping on the train at 5:30, arriving at her IVF clinic at 7:00, hopping on the train again at 7:45, then sidling up to her desk at 9:00. OK, she didn't make it on the dot all the time, but she came pretty close. Today, she recounts those hectic mornings with joy: "Yeah, I was pretty sleep deprived during my treatments. One night, I nodded off right into my dinner plate. But I look back on the experience with warm feelings. IVF was an adventure and, of course, totally worth it." At present, she's a stay-at-home mom with twin boys.

Balancing a job and in-vitro treatments is a tall order, but it can be accomplished. As a cycle heats up, patients are usually required to make near-daily trips to their IVF centers for monitoring between the hours of 7:00 and 9:30 A.M. If you're not a morning person, I urge you to become one at cycle time. Why? The earlier you arrive at your clinic, the less backed up they'll be. Plus, you'll stand a good chance of actually making it to work on time. Sure it may be tempting to hit the snooze button, arrive at the clinic at the last possible minute, then amble into work 45 minutes late. But resist that temptation. On top of everything else, the last thing you need is an irate boss demanding explanations.

And while we're on the topic of bosses, here's the million-dollar question: Should you tell yours about IVF? That really depends on your corporate culture. Businesses—and bosses—run the gamut from the caring to the cantankerous. If you work for a touchy-feely enterprise, it might make sense to give your boss the heads-up so he or she will cut you some slack. If, however, you work for a dog-eat-dog corporation, it's probably wise to stay mum. (After all, you'll be tipping your hand that maternity leave may be next!) Not sure which category your place of employment falls into? Try confiding in a trusted coworker to get his or her take. In the whirl of infertility treatment, it can help to get input from an objective third party.

Now, onto another job-related matter—your workload. Try to stay on top of it. Of course, this may be easier said than done. Cycle side effects include bloating, hot flashes, mood swings, irritability, headaches, and, for some, the frustrating inability to concentrate on simple tasks. Many will get by with mild discomfort, while others will feel like they're clomping through the office with a Hulk-sized case of PMS. Regardless of where you fall on the continuum, understand that your colleagues will probably be pretty clueless about your situation. Be especially kind to yourself, but don't expect them to do the same. Unfortunately, work doesn't stand still for women undergoing IVF. And if your performance starts to suffer, you may get in trouble and that will only serve to increase your consternation. Thus, it's smart to try and do your best work—even if it hurts a little. During those difficult moments, soothe yourself with the knowledge that the unpleasant side effects will pass. And make it a point to pamper yourself each evening with massages, good dinners, and early bedtimes.

And a final tip: For those who simply can't pull off a job and in vitro at the same time—because of scheduling issues or stress—check out the Family and Medical Leave Act (acronym FMLA). This law, passed by Congress in 1993, guarantees up to 12 weeks of unpaid leave to employees coping with serious medical conditions or new babies. To date, more than four million Americans have taken advantage of FMLA to care for a relative or themselves. Of course, there are a few restrictions: To be eligible, candidates must report to a job site with a minimum of 50 employees. They must have worked at least 20 weeks in the past year and been on the payroll for at least a year. In addition, 30 days notice is required. Whether IVFers are eligible for FMLA leave is an ongoing debate, but a number of women *have* successfully made use of it for this purpose. It's important to note, however, that the leave is unpaid. Therefore, the pros of not working should be carefully weighed against the cons of forgoing a paycheck. If FMLA sounds like a solution for you, it's wise to discuss the option with a discreet human resources representative or a lawyer to ensure that you qualify. To learn more, you can also visit the U.S. Department of Labor Web site (www.dol.gov).

On Orientation,
Risks, and Consent Forms

Most IVF centers make a concerted effort to get patients up to speed on in vitro before they undergo it. Smaller practices often offer individual training sessions and/or take-home videos. Larger practices, by contrast, tend to favor one- or two-hour orientations, in which nurses explain the process to incoming "classes" of IVFers. Orientations, how-to videos, and packets of must-read material can feel like school all over again. And some of us might not have liked school too much in the first place. Still, it makes sense to listen and read everything with care. In vitro is a big venture and the more you know, the better prepared you'll be—which *can* have a positive effect on your outcome. Also, resist the temptation to let your partner play hooky during this period. Learning together is an important part of the team-building process—and you'll need each other in the weeks ahead.

Loretta, a 39-year-old sales assistant, recalls her experience: "Understanding IVF was a bit like a jigsaw puzzle. I had some pieces and my husband, Dan, had some others. When we sat down and put them together we had the big picture with a couple of holes. To fill the holes, we asked questions during orientation." Loretta and Dan's strategy is a good one—especially the part about asking questions. During orientation, don't withhold questions for fear of appearing unknowledgeable. Having a firm grasp of the process far outweighs any momentary embarrassment. Besides, the other patients will probably thank you. Chances are they have some of the very same ones!

Next, I wanted to mention an important related issue—IVF consent forms. All practices require patients to sign a series of contractlike forms before treatment can commence. These are often passed out during orientation and serve a few purposes: They spell out the financial arrangement, outline what couples can expect during the course of their treatment, and, perhaps most importantly, inform them of the risks commonly associated with in vitro fertilization.

So you won't be surprised down the road, let's go over the major risks:

Multiple Gestation and/or the Need for Selective Reduction

A major concern of many IVFers is that they'll get pregnant with two, three, even four babies. Fact: Roughly 36 percent of all women who undergo the process give birth to multiples. When I heard, "We think you're pregnant with twins," it was music to my ears. However, multiple gestation poses some very serious health risks for mother and babies—and those risks get increasingly pronounced with each additional fetus. Problems include troubled pregnancies, premature delivery, and a high incidence of birth defects and developmental problems (such as cerebral palsy). Such worries are real and cannot be wished away.

For that reason, REs counsel patients to think long and hard about the number of embryos to transfer. To make an informed decision IVFers will also need to do some soul-searching regarding selective reduction. In this outpatient procedure, performed with the aid of ultrasound, a needle containing a special chemical is injected into one of the fetuses. (Doctors do a number of tests in an attempt to select the one that is already the most at risk.) Its heart is then stopped and, over time, the fetus is reabsorbed into the tissue of the uterus. The decision to undergo selective reduction is a highly personal one. Still, many IVFers choose reduction so that the remaining baby or babies stand a better chance of thriving. (These important topics will be explored in greater depth in Chapter 9.)

Miscarriage and Ectopic Pregnancies

Sadly, about 25 percent of all pregnancies end in miscarriage, but with in vitro those numbers rise to about 30 percent. In addition, IVF increases the chances of ectopic pregnancies (when embryos develop outside the uterus, usually in the fallopian tubes) from 1 percent to roughly 2 percent. Why is this the case? Even though embryos are placed in the uterus, they occasionally drift into the fallopian tubes and get trapped there. This problem is especially prevalent in women with partially blocked tubes because embryos tend to get "hemmed in" by dilations and scar tissue. Ectopic pregnancies, which almost always result in miscarriage, can be dangerous if the embryos are left to develop to the point of rupturing the tubes. It's essential to understand, however, that the risks of ectopic pregnancies are higher among IVFers because a large number of women with tubal issues undergo it.

Ovarian Hyperstimulation Syndrome

The goal of superovulatory drugs is to produce multiple eggs. As a result, women's ovaries usually get temporarily enlarged, occasionally to three or four times their normal size. This causes bloating, fluid retention, and, in about 1 to 2 percent of patients, a problem called ovarian hyperstimulation syndrome (OHSS). Bad cases of OHSS can lead to canceled cycles and/or hospital stays to ensure the patient doesn't experience blood clots, twisted ovaries, or kidney or liver damage. Although the condition sounds scary, it's comforting to know that all IVFers receive frequent OHSS monitoring in the form of estradiol blood tests and ultrasounds—two effective safeguards that protect most women from ever developing it. That being said, the condition can and does occur, especially in patients with polycystic ovarian syndrome. (For more information see Chapter 9.)

Infection

There is about a one in a thousand chance that a pelvic infection will occur as a result of egg retrieval. A small percentage to be sure, but worth a mention. Most of the reported infections have been mild, but a handful have been severe enough to merit surgery. Most REs wisely prescribe antibiotics around retrieval time to reduce the risk.

Ovarian and Breast Cancer

The link between cancer and IVF has been the subject of much debate and controversy over the years. One study demonstrated a slightly higher rate of ovarian and breast cancer among women who used a lot of superovulatory drugs, while another study showed no increase at all. Some research even suggests that IVF is beneficial because achieving a pregnancy tends to slightly reduce the occurrence of ovarian cancer. Bottom line? The jury's still out. There's no compelling proof that IVFers face a greater threat of developing cancer. But twenty or thirty years down the road, who knows? Women considering in vitro should be aware of the issue so they can factor it into their decision.

In a nutshell, the risks associated with in vitro appear to be no greater than those faced by women undergoing any number of routine medical procedures. The operative word here is *appear*. Because in vitro is such a new science, problematic outcomes have not yet been compiled and widely studied. Thus, each factor listed above should be considered with a critical eye. If you'd like to learn more, I suggest you speak with your RE and spend a few hours gathering facts on the Internet. There's certainly a lot of anecdotal information out there, both pro and con. When it comes to risks, everyone has a different comfort level. No doubt a few readers will even opt out of IVF because they simply cannot make peace with all the unknowns. That's certainly valid. The important thing is to educate yourself on key issues before embarking on a cycle. To help you do that, here are some other priority issues to mull over:

- How many eggs should be fertilized?

- How many embryos should be transferred?

- In the case of multiples, is selective reduction an acceptable option?

- Should ISCI and assisted hatching be employed to promote pregnancy?

- Should "extra" high-quality embryos be frozen, discarded, or donated to other couples?

- Should poor-quality embryos be discarded or donated to scientific research?

Seem like some big questions? They are. While it's true that most IVF consent forms must be completed *before* you cycle, they're seldom demanded on the spot. My advice: Take the paperwork home, read and discuss it with your partner, then return to your center at a later date to sign them. And if you have lingering queries, don't stand on ceremony. Call a knowledgeable person at your practice and ask him or her to explain your options in layman language. (A lawyer isn't necessary unless you're making use of an egg donor or gestational surrogate.) Know, too, that at least one of these decisions—how many embryos to transfer—can and should be deferred until *later* in your cycle when you have more to go on. Nevertheless, you and your mate should work together to develop a comfortable response to each question. Sound overwhelming? Support is on the way in the form of Chapter 9. It will help to focus your thinking by providing much-needed background information. In the meantime, keep reading to learn about a few other pre-cycle orders of business.

Money Matters

The gist of this section can be summed up in a single sentence: *Know exactly how much your IVF cycle will cost and set aside the money to pay for it.* Although a few clinics offer long-term payment plans, the majority demand payment in full before the delivery of services (unless, of course, you're one of the lucky ones with insurance). At my practice, for example, I put $1,000 down at orientation, another $2,000 down at the start of my cycle, then ponied up the balance— about $10,000—the day before my retrieval. Since I hate parting with cash, it stung less to have my husband write the checks. If you, too, plan on paying by check, take a peek at your bank account balance to make sure the expenditure will clear. If you're planning on using a credit card, call MasterCard or Visa to make sure your line of credit is sufficient. Unfortunately, there's seldom wiggle room for late payments. As much as your IVF center cares about you, they're running a business. That means if the monies due aren't paid on time, your cycle will likely be canceled. Therefore, IVFers are wise to have their financial ducks in a row *before* beginning treatment.

And a final tip: Make sure to ask your IVF center about their refund policies. Occasionally cycles get canceled before completion and money is due back to IVFers. For that reason, it's best to know what to expect to ensure that you receive the reimbursement due you.

Getting Medications

Another pre-cycle order of business is making a plan to get all of your medications in a timely manner—preferably at a reduced price.

The fertility drugs you'll need are expensive, costing between $2,000 and $4,000 per cycle. Thus, it's pretty tempting to wait until the eleventh hour to purchase them. After all, cycles do get canceled. That certainly makes sense, but there's a caveat: Don't postpone the purchase too long. Andi, a 30-year-old actress, learned that lesson the hard way: "During my first IVF cycle I was pretty casual about stuff. When the nurse called to tell me it was time to start my super-ovulatory drugs, I was excited. There was only one problem. When shot time rolled around at 9:00 P.M., I couldn't find my Gonal F. I had a prescription, but I'd forgotten to buy it! That had me calling every 24-hour pharmacy in town—none had it! In a blue panic, I phoned my RE. He sent me over to the clinic, where I was greeted by a nurse. In the parking lot, she slipped me a few bottles that she pulled out of their secret stash. Covert meetings, idling cars, sweaty palms—it felt like a spy thriller. Yes, I got the shot, but not without a lot of aggravation. The next day, I made a trip to a pharmacy that specialized in fertility drugs and bought everything I needed."

Andi's late-night adventure illustrates a point: Fertility drugs are seldom in stock at standard drugstores. They have to be special-ordered, which can take a week or more. For that reason, it's wise to have a conversation with your RE regarding the best timetable and method of obtaining them well before your cycle begins. Some IVF centers have on-site drug dispensaries; others work with a local pharmacy that makes it a point to keep these drugs in stock. But even with these options available, it's not a bad idea to widen the circle and comparison shop. In-vitro medications are also available though a host of online and mail-order pharmacies—many offering considerable discounts. That means if you do your homework, you could save several hundred bucks. Just be sure to thoroughly check out such brokers to make sure they're on the up and up (most are).

And beware of folks hawking cut-rate fertility drugs in Internet chat rooms. Some may be running scams and/or trafficking in questionable merchandise. Believe it or not, *there is* a thriving black market out there. Sure, everyone loves a great deal. However, just like a side of beef that's fallen off a truck, there's no guarantee that you'll get a quality product. How will you know, for example, that the meds have been properly stored and haven't exceeded their expiration dates? How will you know they're even the real McCoy? My opinion, for what it's worth, is to simply say no to drugs from questionable sources. That includes well-intentioned IVFers who want to give you their leftovers. No doubt it's a generous act, but who needs the added worry of wondering whether their fertility meds will actually work?

And two final hints: After purchasing your meds, take a careful inventory to make sure you received everything you were supposed to. Even the best pharmacist can make mistakes. Second, don't forget to submit all claims to your insurance company. Even when nothing else is covered, sometimes meds are! And we're not talking chump change here.

Cycle Do's and Don'ts

While researching this book, I spoke with a number of reproductive endocrinologists. All of them were wise and dedicated. And all of them agreed on the basic tenets of an effective treatment plan. None, however, concurred on every single detail. Give me a hundred REs and they'll give you a hundred slightly different versions of the best way to go about in vitro. One, for example, may ban caffeine of any kind and think yoga is a great mid-cycle stress reliever. Meanwhile, a colleague will opine that it's perfectly fine to down a cup of coffee or two, but may worry that an ambitious yoga position might twist enlarged ovaries. My point: Do's and Don'ts are as individual as the doctors who issue them. Therefore, it's essential to speak with yours to get a full rundown on the behaviors that will promote a successful cycle. After all, your choice of that doctor is a vote of confidence in his or her methodology and opinions.

First and foremost, be sure to discuss any medications you're on. When Sandy, a 39-year-old nurse practitioner, met with her doctor to plan her upcoming cycle, he felt strongly that she should try to do it without the Prozac she takes for depression. (While there is no evidence to suggest that antidepressants affect developing fetuses, most REs counsel against them.) Sandy recalls: "The hardest part of in vitro was getting off the Prozac that I'd been on for two years. I knew it would be hard so I planned accordingly. A few months before treatment I worked with my therapist to reduce my dosage a bit each week and by cycle time I was completely off. It was tough, but not as tough as I thought. Now, I'm thrilled to have a baby, and I'm back on my meds." Miranda's RE had an equally strong opinion regarding her medication—by all means, take it. "I give myself heparin injections for a blood-clotting disorder," this 29-year-old librarian told me. "My doctor was crystal clear: Take every shot of heparin or IVF won't work. Needless to say, I followed her orders to the letter."

Following your doctor's orders to the letter, as Miranda did, is the right strategy. Not only will it help ensure a healthier cycle, it will keep you from wandering down the obsessive road of what-ifs. *What if I didn't have six cups of coffee each day during treatment? What if I didn't bike 25 miles that afternoon? What if I didn't drink that bottle of wine to calm me down?* Although it's very possible that none of these behaviors will have any effect on your treatment, my personal take is that it's best to err on the side of caution. That way, you'll know you did everything in your power to maximize your chances—regardless of whether your cycle succeeds or fails. "I did in vitro three times," reports Peggy, a 40-year-old illustrator. "The first two times, I didn't do anything special. The third time around, though, I rethought things. My new plan was to treat my body as if it were *already* pregnant. That meant early to bed. That meant no booze. That meant taking a prenatal vitamin and eating the right foods. I can't say my new philosophy made a difference. But I *can* say that I got pregnant."

Peggy's approach to her third cycle of IVF is smart. After all, if it goes well, you'll soon be pregnant anyway. So why not get a head start on healthy behaviors? The majority of REs agree that the following lists of do's and don'ts make sense during cycle time.

Let's start with the "do's" . . .

1. DO make sure all your requisite tests are out of the way, even those that seem pretty silly. If you fail to take even one of them, there's a good chance your cycle will be canceled.

2. DO take a prenatal vitamin and folic acid before and during treatment. These will help ensure the development of a healthy fetus—or two!

3. DO eat a balanced diet. Your body is going through a lot and you want to keep it well nourished.

4. DO drink lots of fluids. Dehydration can make it harder for nurses to draw blood from your veins.

5. DO speak with your RE about sexual activity. (For more information on the topic see Chapter 9.)

6. DO get in touch with your practice if you have questions during your treatment. Getting answers will help you remain relaxed and centered.

7. DO inform your RE if you are sick. While mild illnesses are not cause for concern, a very high fever *can* have a deleterious effect on developing embryos. In addition, an outbreak of herpes can also be an issue.

8. DO go to bed early. A good night's sleep will empower you to cope with the demands of early-morning treatments.

9. DO continue moderate exercise, such as walking or light workouts. Keeping your body active—but not overactive—will likely have a calming effect on your mind.

10. DO consider keeping a journal of your IVF journey. Many women—and men—find that privately writing about their experiences gives them a safe place to explore feelings.

11. DO pamper yourself. Movies, country drives, good books, and favorite tunes will help you maintain a positive frame of mind.

12. DO let your partner pamper you. Allowing your significant other to cater to you during this challenging period will probably make him feel better, too.

Now, on to some pesky "don'ts":

1. DON'T eat "risky" foods such as sushi, greasy-spoon grub, or unpasteurized cheeses such as Brie or Stilton. Although unlikely, a bad case of food poisoning can end an otherwise promising cycle.

2. DON'T diet. IVF calls for your undivided attention and strength. Dieting during treatment will only add to your stress and, down the road, will deprive a developing fetus of essential nutrition.

3. DON'T drink more than one or two caffeinated beverages a day. Although there is not conclusive evidence to suggest that caffeine affects fertility, it doesn't hurt to be conservative.

4. DON'T drink more than one alcoholic beverage per day, if that. A glass of wine to calm you down may be permissible (ask your RE), but too much booze can cloud your thinking, make you depressed, and/or cause you to miss your appointments.

5. DON'T smoke cigarettes or do recreational drugs. Research shows that cigarettes, marijuana, and cocaine are all bad news for developing babies.

6. DON'T take any medications without speaking to your doctor first. As I previously mentioned, certain prescription and over-the-counter drugs—even ibuprofen, adult-dosage aspirin, or a flu shot—can have an impact on success.

7. DON'T take any natural herbs. Herbal remedies in the form of pills, tinctures, or teas affect metabolism and may reduce your ability to get pregnant.

8. DON'T run excessively or overdo the exercise. Jogging, especially long distances, can twist oversized ovaries. So can intensive workouts. Thus, it's imperative to speak with your RE about any and all physical activities.

9. DON'T indulge in saunas, Jacuzzis, hot tubs, or very hot baths—that goes for both partners! Heat can reduce fertility, particularly sperm counts.

10. DON'T have sex without a condom or a diaphragm. Although there is no evidence that suggests getting pregnant on Lupron is dangerous to fetuses, it's wise to play it safe by using birth control. Believe me, it *can happen*—even with a diagnosis of infertility.

11. DON'T travel too far from your IVF center (unless you have to). If something goes wrong, you'll want to be in close proximity to your practice.

12. DON'T take on extra projects. Undergoing IVF is challenge enough.

13. DON'T make dates with difficult friends or family members. The last thing you need is more agitation.

14. DON'T retreat from the land of the living. Yes, you should take it easy. But try to resist the temptation to cut yourself off from key loved ones and touchstones. Depriving yourself of these nurturing forces may cause you to feel isolated.

15. DON'T beat up on yourself during those moments you're feeling less than positive. Occasional negative vibes are normal and won't affect the outcome of a cycle.

While we're on the topics of do's and don'ts, let me slip in a maybe: acupuncture. A staple in China for 2,000 years, acupuncture is gaining well-deserved respect in the Western world. In fact, a recent German study found that IVF success rates were boosted by 50 percent when a few sessions of acupuncture were added to the mix. The study was a small one, but a number of REs are becoming true believers. Some are even recommending the therapy to their patients. What is it? This ancient practice involves placing hair-thin needles at key points in the skin. How does it work? The theory holds that the needles stimulate the autonomic nervous system, which helps control the muscles and glands, thereby rendering the lining of the uterus more receptive to incoming embryos.

Fertility Fact: A recent study suggests that nonsmokers are twice as likely to have success with IVF as those who smoke.

Jill Blakeway, a licensed acupuncturist in New York City, has developed an expertise in treating IVFers: "I work with many women undergoing in vitro fertilization. When I do, I always speak with a patient's reproductive endocrinologist, then coordinate my treatments with key points in their in-vitro cycle. My patients tend to enjoy their sessions. Many find them relaxing and some even comment they feel warm and fuzzy when they're over." She adds, "We're not exactly sure how it works, but it's certainly getting results for me!" My friend Greta would concur. Jill treated her following two failed rounds of IVF. "When I didn't have success with my first couple of cycles, I decided to try acupuncture on a whim," shares Greta, a 41-year-old psychiatrist. "I can't state with authority that it made the difference, but I have a hunch it did. My baby shower is next week!" If you're interested in pursuing this course of treatment, there's one caveat: Be sure to pick a licensed acupuncturist with direct experience in infertility. Prices range from $50 to $100 a session.

A Final To-Do List

Well, as promised, we've certainly covered a lot of ground in this chapter. I hope it has provided clear strategies to help you feel fit and prepared for your IVF journey. But are you really ready to cycle? To find out, take a few minutes to peruse the items on the following to-do list. Then, put a checkmark beside each task you've completed.

☐ 1. I have a thorough understanding of the IVF process.

☐ 2. I have had a frank discussion with my RE in which he or she has informed me of my basic chances of succeeding with one cycle.

☐ 3. I have decided on the optimal time to schedule my IVF cycle. I have figured out a plan for balancing work and treatments. My partner's calendar is also clear and he is on board to help me.

☐ 4. I have been told of the risks associated with IVF, including the very real possibility of multiples.

☐ 5. I have had a discussion with my partner regarding how many embryos to transfer, as well as our position regarding selective reduction.

☐ 6. I have the money set aside for treatments.

☐ 7. I know what medications I need and where to get them.

☐ 8. I have discussed cycle do's and don'ts with my RE and am prepared to abide by his or her suggestions.

☐ 9. I have planned for the possibility that a single cycle of IVF won't work and I have a contingency plan in place.

☐ 10. I have planned for the possibility that a single cycle of IVF may well work and I'll soon be pregnant.

Did you place a check beside each and every item? If so, you're all set for IVF. If not, it's a good idea to go back and do a little more thinking. No doubt it would be nice if these logistical and emotionally charged issues just melted away so we wouldn't have to deal with them head-on. But ignoring them is probably a bad plan. My advice? Sit down with your partner and hash things out together. Teamwork and discussion and thoughtful choices will help empower you to have a great cycle. "Thinking and thinking about IVF made our brains hurt so much we'd spend some evenings watching cheesy reruns of *Three's Company* and *Who's the Boss?* just to recover," laughs Talisa, a 30-year-old freelance editor. "But all that careful planning paid off. We knew just what to expect when the treatments kicked in."

Chapter 9

Questions and Answers About Your Cycle

ॐ

Welcome to the Club

With the exception of a brief stint as a Brownie at the tender age of seven, I have a tendency to be pretty club resistant. Girl Scouts, sororities, book groups, you name it—I never belonged to a one. Nothing against them, I'm just not much of a joiner. Then came two years of failed attempts to get pregnant and my unwitting initiation into the infertility club. I have to admit, initially, I kicked and screamed. As Groucho Marx famously remarked, "I don't want to be part of a club that will accept me as a member." I wanted to be "normal." I wanted to have a baby the good old-fashioned way, without intervention.

But, in the midst of my quest for a child, a surprising thing happened: I stepped into the bustling waiting room of an IVF center. First, I surveyed the surroundings. *Hmmm. Appealing shades of maroon and mauve with tasteful flower paintings.* Next, I scanned the faces. All around me were women—some in carefully pressed business suits, others in jeans and t-shirts. Some read magazines. Several chatted in clutches. A number looked up and smiled. One woman with knitting needles leaned over, squeezed my hand, and said, "You're new here, aren't you?" I managed a shy "yes" to which she responded, "Then Welcome—welcome to the club!" *Club.* She invoked the c-word.

Yet this time it felt absolutely right. Her friendly words soothed my jangled nerves and made me feel at home. And in the weeks that followed, the two of us—along with a bunch of 7:30 A.M. regulars—formed a pretty tight bond. We talked. Supported one another. Even laughed. At long last, I'd found a group that I was proud to join: Kim and Yasmine and Caroline, Dorie and Amanda. Here was a lively, diligent, diverse community of women facing the challenge of infertility and doing something about it. Women who are probably a lot like you.

This is perhaps the most important chapter in the entire book. Its purpose? To provide background on what's to come during your actual cycle—from the first shot of Lupron to the culminating pregnancy test. Because there are so many topics to cover, I've arranged things a bit differently from the previous chapters. This one is written in question-and-answer form to provide concise information on the myriad issues that may be weighing on your mind. To write it, I reflected upon my own IVF experience, recalling all the questions that I had, including: *How do I keep track of my protocol? Will I be able to manage the shots? What's egg retrieval like? How many embryos should I transfer? What's the risk of miscarriage?* This section may be read in its entirety or grazed over with an eye toward addressing your most pressing concerns. Either way, it's my intention to offer an honest account of what to expect during a cycle—from one member of the club to another.

Commonly Asked Questions About Embarking on an IVF Cycle

Before starting a cycle, you may have a few lingering big-picture questions. I thought it fitting to begin this chapter with some information to help ensure a smooth journey.

How Do I Keep Track of My Protocol?

Most clinics provide a photocopied calendar of sorts for their patients to follow. This outlines the basic IVF timeline and sometimes includes information on specific medications and dosages. Keep it near at hand. It's important. That being said, no protocol is written in stone. Yes, REs can conjecture about how you'll respond to specific meds, but they can't know for certain. As a result, dosages and timetables can and do change on a daily basis. For example, if your eggs are growing slower than expected, your doctor may up your dose of superovulatory drugs and move your retrieval from Friday to Saturday. That's to be expected. The best REs are skilled in the art of improvisation.

Still, sudden tweaks to a treatment plan can be unsettling to patients. To become more comfortable with the concept, try thinking of your cycle as a road trip. You know where you want to go—Pregnancyville—but the journey there might not go exactly as planned. It may require detours. It may take a few days longer than anticipated. That's fine. The important thing is to focus on your destination *and* remain utterly meticulous about tracking your route. What do I mean? During the egg-ripening phase, it's customary for nurses to phone patients in late afternoon to announce daily dosages. My recommendation? Write down exactly what they say *right away* in some kind of log. You'd be surprised how quickly numbers can get confused when they're not committed to paper. And a couple mistakes can compromise a cycle.

Different types of record-keeping techniques work for different types of people. Mandy bought one of those large desk calendars, filling in her tentative cycle in pencil. Then, when things changed, she used her trusty eraser and made corrections. Carol jotted everything down in her beloved Filofax. Amy relied on a dry-erase board. Liv used a journal, color coding medications and adding notes about how she was feeling. As for me, I fired up my computer and created a gridlike calendar. On it, I entered every office visit and drug dosage as well as the projected date of my egg retrieval, transfer, and pregnancy test. When variables changed—no problem!—I simply edited the document.

What's the very best way to keep tabs on your treatment plan? That's for you to decide. The trick is to be especially exacting, even if that means playing against type. In everyday life, it's great to be laid back and loosey-goosey, but IVF calls for almost militaristic adherence to doctors' orders. Cassandra, a 30-year-old playwright, shared her secret: "I don't like fine print. When I play Boggle or Monopoly, I make up my own rules. So in vitro was a bit of a challenge for me. To make it work, I invented this character named Mrs. Bartlebine and kind of channeled her. Mrs. Bartlebine was totally uptight. She wrote everything down in a spiral notebook. She made her husband double-check her work. After awhile, it became our little joke. I'd announce, 'Mrs. B. is awaiting her injections,' and my hubby would come running in to help make sure I did them just right."

Will I See My RE a Lot During My Cycle?

That really depends on the type of IVF practice you've chosen. If it's a small one with a single RE, chances are you'll see that doctor during most of your office visits. (As a general rule of thumb, doctors do ultrasounds as well as procedures, while nurses handle blood tests, record-keeping, and afternoon phone calls regarding dosages.) If, however, you've selected a practice that has several REs, it's very likely they'll pool resources. That means that your sonograms—and quite possibly your egg retrieval and embryo transfer—may be performed by *other* doctors on the staff.

That was certainly true in my case. Following my initial consultation, I saw my RE of record very little. At first, this alarmed me a bit. *Poof! It was almost as if he up and disappeared! Where the heck was this esteemed, expensive expert?* I thought. Then I took the time to find out how the clinic operated: Twice weekly, the five REs met and decided together how each patient's treatment should proceed. In addition, I learned that my own doctor checked all my blood tests and ultrasounds, then told the nurse what my daily dosages of fertility drugs should be. Sure, the nurse called me, but my RE was the one driving my treatment plan. I have to say my little fact-finding mission made me feel better. I actually liked the idea of several doctors weighing in on my case. The way I figured it, five heads were better than one. Of course, it's important to understand that every practice is run differently. Therefore, it probably makes sense to find out how yours goes about divvying up its duties. Chances are a thorough explanation of the process will help bring you peace of mind.

Can We Have Sex During IVF?

For some couples, maintaining an active sex life during in vitro is desirable. It helps them feel alive; it helps them feel normal. Others will place lovemaking at the bottom of their to-do list. Basia, a 33-year-old business consultant, told me, "I was so pumped up on hormones and stress, a roll in the hay was the farthest thing from my mind." Either way, it's wise to have a candid conversation with your RE about intercourse during IVF, including specific times when it is and isn't advisable. No, I'm not passing the buck here. It's simply that different doctors have different opinions. For example, some believe that sexual activity prior to the HCG shot is a good thing because it stimulates hormones that subtly improve implantation and helps men maintain a "fresher" sperm sample. In fact, a few even prescribe it! On the other hand, many REs worry that sex after retrieval can trigger cervical infections or compromise the uterine lining. While the jury is still out on some of these theories, the best course of action is to ask your own doctor.

Fertility Fact: 1980 is the date of the first baby born from an IVF protocol that included superovulatory drugs.

Now, a word about birth control. If you do have sex, be sure to use barrier protection (a condom or diaphragm). Although it may sound ridiculous, even couples diagnosed with severe infertility can get pregnant naturally during their cycle. *I know, I know, the whole point of in vitro is to have a baby so what's wrong with that?* Here goes: That developing embryo may be exposed to a host of fertility meds in utero. While there is no evidence to suggest that drugs such as Lupron pose any threat, there's no conclusive research to prove they don't. Therefore, it's wise to play it safe by using protection.

Any Tips for Making My Morning Trips to the IVF Clinic More Pleasant?

First, drink plenty of water before anticipated blood tests. Hydrating your body will make it easier for the nurses to locate your veins and draw blood. Second, to avoid patient logjam, try arriving extra early. Third, always be prepared for a bit of waiting. To pass time, I recommend high-interest reading material—newspapers, glossy magazines, potboilers. (Likely, you won't be able to focus on the likes of *Ulysses!*)

Some women bring crossword puzzles, knitting, even Gameboys. Others bring their partners. I have to admit mine came in pretty handy. He escorted me to as many appointments as he could. Having him beside me soothed my nerves and reminded me that we were in this together. And if the appointment went quickly, we'd have time to stop at our favorite diner for scrambled eggs and bacon before heading off in opposite directions to work.

Commonly Asked Questions About Step 1: Suppression and Developing Eggs

The suppression and egg-development phase encompasses the first two-and-a-half to three weeks of an IVF cycle. During this time frame, most IVFers receive Lupron to suppress normal ovulation. Then, when their periods arrive—which may be scant—they begin superovulatory drugs to stimulate the maturation of numerous eggs. Let's take a look at some questions you may have about this important step.

Mixing Meds and Giving Myself Shots Sounds Tricky. Will I Ever Get the Hang of It?

A resounding yes! When it comes to in vitro, patients are required to mix and administer their own medications. This responsibility has stricken fear into the heart of many an IVFer—myself included. I still remember returning home from the pharmacy with a bag bursting with fertility medication (price tag, $3,000). I lined up the contents on my coffee table. It's an understatement to say there were a lot of little bottles. One was filled with a clear fluid; this was the Lupron. A few dozen contained white powder; this was the superovulatory medication. A few dozen more contained saline solution; this would be used to dissolve the powder into a liquid for injections. In addition, there were pads of gauze and alcohol wipes. And, last but not least, two big bundles of needles. My initial reaction went something like this—*Help!!!* I immediately flashed back to tenth-grade chemistry class in which almost all of my experiments failed. Mixing and measuring was clearly not my forte. I practically started hyperventilating. Then, I did what I always do in times of crisis—I took a deep breath and talked myself down by saying, *If hundreds of thousands of other women can handle this responsibility, so can I.*

I was right. In a few short days, I had the shots down to a science. And dare I say it, I even began to look forward to the nightly ritual of mixing and administering my injections. I'd put on a favorite CD, rouse my husband from his computer, then the two of us would spend some quality shot-time together. First, I'd inject the Lupron, then I'd follow it up with the superovulatory drugs. As it turns out, mixing was a breeze—amounting to little more than injecting a syringe filled with saline into the bottle of powder to convert it to liquid, then sucking it up into a different syringe for the actual injection. I won't go into the nitty-gritty of administering medications here—that's best left to your IVF nurse. However, I do want to offer a few tips that I picked up from the many women I interviewed for this book. So here goes . . .

First, be absolutely anal when it comes to medications. Make sure you know exactly how much you're supposed to take. And when you're certain you've got the measurement down, ask your partner to double-check your calculations. You can't be too careful. Believe it or not, many a cycle has been blown by an IVFer who accidentally took too much or too little. Second, practice by giving shots to an orange. (It won't mind!) Simply ask your doctor to include a few extra needles and bottles of saline along with your prescription. Then, "play IVF" by injecting the fluid into the orange. The needle should enter it swiftly at a ninety degree angle, kind of like a dart. Third, don't be thrown by unfamiliar lingo such as *ampules* ("amps")—this is just a fancy name for the tiny glass bottles that house the meds; or *sharps*—a nickname for needles; or *cubic centimeters* ("CCs")—the metric measurement most often used for IVF shots. And speaking of shots, have I mentioned there are two varieties:

✣ **Subcutaneous Injections:** These "short" shots require half-inch needles. They get injected just under the skin, usually in the thigh or abdomen. This size needle is used to administer Lupron, Gonal F, Follistim, Bravelle, and Repronex.

❧ **Intramuscular Injections:** These "long" shots require one-and-a-half-inch needles. They get injected deep into muscle, usually in the upper-outer quadrant of the butt. This size needle is used for HCG and progesterone. Although a few IVFers are skilled enough to contort their bodies to administer their own shots, most rely on their partner to do it for them.

Now that you've learned some medical lingo, here are some random tips to help you master the process:

1. Unless your doctor tells you otherwise, make it a point to administer your injections at the same general time each day. Most often that's the evening, but some IVFers take both morning and evening shots.

2. Put on your favorite tunes to create a relaxing atmosphere.

3. Wash your hands with soap and water before getting started.

4. Know thy needles. Make sure you're using the proper size for the job. Using the "short" needle to administer HCG, for example, will greatly reduce its effectiveness.

5. Cleanse the injection site with alcohol. Pinching or rubbing ice over it may help deaden the pain. Some folks even use Anbesol.

6. Never touch the tip of a needle—that will contaminate it. Use each needle only once. On top of being unsanitary, pre-used needles have dull points, which will make injections more painful.

7. Alternate injection sites each night. For example, if you gave yourself Lupron in your right thigh, switch to your left for the following shot.

8. Don't toss your needles in the trash—they're dangerous! If you were not provided with a plastic "sharps" bin, place them in a

sealed coffee can or detergent bottle. Then return them to your IVF clinic for proper disposal.

9. Store your medication in a safe place away from the sun, pouncing cats, children, and nosy visitors. And remember, Lupron gets refrigerated after use.

10. Treat yourself to a take-out meal, candy bar, or favorite video after shot time to congratulate yourself on a job well done.

Last but not least, if you're confused about the optimal location for an intramuscular injection, bring in a pair of panties and ask a nurse to cut out two holes to show you. Then, at shot time, put them on! Another solution is to ask her to draw marker circles on your skin. Nancy, a 32-year-old marketing executive, recalls: "An IVF nurse drew targets to indicate where my progesterone injections should go. Later that day, during a work meeting, I thought about those double bull's-eyes on my butt and burst out laughing. Of course, I couldn't share the source of my amusement with my coworkers." Although it may sound a bit unorthodox, rest assured, most nurses are skilled at such graphics. They're also pretty unflappable, which brings me to my final point: If you have any questions, big or small, don't stand on ceremony. Call your IVF center right away for guidance. Don't let a little embarrassment put your cycle in jeopardy!

But What If I'm Deathly Afraid of Needles?

Almost everyone has a phobia or two. For me, it's mice. If I spy one, I'm up on a tabletop before you can say "exterminator." For my friend Patsy, it's heights. And for Melinda, a 40-year-old software developer, it was needles. Let me give you some background. This was a woman who hiked the Andes, ate every kind of sushi, and parasailed! Nothing fazed her, it seemed, with the exception of injections. But that phobia was a biggie—forcing her to postpone infertility treatment for five long years. Finally, at the age of 38, she ventured to an RE who leveled with her: IVF was the answer, but if she didn't act quickly, it might be too late. True, she hated needles, but she really loved kids. So she screwed up every ounce of courage and guess what? The shots weren't nearly as bad as she'd built them up to be. The truth is that reality seldom competes with a rich imagination. Epilogue: Today she's mom to rambunctious triplets, comforting them through *their* many vaccinations. It seems the student has become the teacher!

OK, truth time: Subcutaneous shots—the half-inch needles—really, truly, barely hurt at all. Intramuscular injections—the inch-and-a-half needles–sometimes sting a little, but they're nothing compared to a stubbed toe or leg cramp. And I'm sure you handle those just fine. Plus, shots are pretty darn safe. Each week millions of people receive them safely and soundly. So what's all the fuss about? Franklin Roosevelt said, "We have nothing to fear, but fear itself." That little sound bite can certainly be applied to the topic of injections. Most folks who hate them are afraid of the *idea*, which sets off a panic response. This panic response makes their hearts race, palms sweat, and thinking blur. Thus, what they come to fear is not so much the shot as their response to the *suggestion* of a shot.

Ring any bells? Quite possibly you're one of many, many people who dread injections. If that's the case, cut yourself some slack. Everybody, even Wonder Woman, is afraid of something. But how do you get around this little roadblock? A good starting place is to fess up about your phobia. Coming out of the closet and talking about it may relieve some of the pressure. Be candid with your RE or nurse. Chances are they're well versed in this fear and have some tricks up their sleeve for easing the process. One piece of advice *I* can offer is to act quickly and decisively. The more you prolong the injection, the longer you'll experience the panic response. Some find that a countdown of *5, 4, 3, 2, 1, go!* motivates their arm to act. Others rely on deep breathing exercises to slow their heart rates and calm their minds. Still others recruit partners or trusted friends to do the deed for them (medical experience is a plus). While the recruit is administering the shot, your mind's eye can be conjuring up images of a Maui sunset—so what if you've never been there!

The point is to locate a strategy that works for you. And if all else fails, consider hiring a nurse from your IVF practice. Many moonlight as expert shot-givers and will be more than happy to stop by your home after hours to do your injections lickety-split. The going rate is about $25 a shot (for a total of $500 or so). For most needle-phobes, that's a small price to pay for peace of mind and the chance for a baby. Bridget agrees. This 37-year-old ad sales rep recalls: "I just couldn't bring myself to do the shots. And my husband was a wimp, too. So we hired a nurse to come over every night at 7:00. I can't say it was fun, but it wasn't too bad. The knowledge that a trained profes-sional was doing my injections eased my mind plus we really bonded. I even gave her a nickname—Quick-Draw McGraw! When my preg-nancy test came back positive she got a big hug. I couldn't have done it without her!"

What Happens If I Make a Mistake on a Dosage?

Medication mix-ups can and do happen—even to the most meticu-lous IVFers. In fact, a typically cautious friend of mine mismeasured a single dosage of the superovulatory drug Follistim and ended up giving herself five times the prescribed amount! (Fortunately, doc-tors were able to compensate for the error by giving her less in the next couple days.) As mentioned earlier, make every effort to be su-per careful with every measurement. But if you think or know you made a mistake, don't panic. *Do* call your RE right away to report the details. Perhaps it's no big deal. And if it is, your doctor may be able to make an appropriate adjustment to save your cycle.

How Will the Medications Make Me Feel?

Now that we've spent a little time on dosages, let's take a moment to talk about how these medications will make you feel. I interviewed dozens of women for this book and can report that the range of fertility-drug side effects is wider than the Grand Canyon. Lee, a 31-year-old personal assistant, said, "I didn't feel too bad at all. Just a lit-tle tired and headachy—kind of like a very mild case of the flu." Laurie-Ann, a 38-year-old wedding planner, reports, "I was functional, but felt a little out of sorts. And my concentration was off: I'd sit down to read a book and feel like I was slipping right off the page." Caro-line, a 29-year-old homemaker, remembers, "I was really, really emo-tional—extreme highs, extreme lows. It was like my emotions were turned up to 11." Meanwhile, Lena, a 41-year-old textile designer, sampled everything on the menu: "I was really bloated, to the point that I couldn't button my pants. I had hot flashes, nausea, and a throbbing head. I was moody and distracted. And maybe it was my imagination, but I could have sworn that I felt my ovaries expanding. It was like I had the worst case of PMS on the planet."

Needless to say Lena was not a happy camper. That is, until she muddled through treatments and ended up pregnant. For most, the symptoms associated with the IVF drug regimen are annoying. For a minority, they border on temporarily debilitating. What accounts for the difference? For one thing, some women take three or even five times the dosage of superovulatory drugs that their counterparts do. This can have an impact. But a bigger factor is how an individual's body responds to treatment. As a general rule of thumb, those who produce the most eggs—say, 20, 30, or more—get hit the hardest with symptoms. Why? The large number of growing eggs trigger the production of hormones with a host of unpleasant side effects, not unlike those experienced by Lena. These "strong responders," as they are often referred to, are also at the greatest risk for developing ovarian hyperstimulation syndrome (see following section to learn more).

Regardless of whether your symptoms rate a 1 or 10 on the Richter scale, it's important to take very good care of yourself during cycle time. Just as folks with colds or flus rest up, so, too, should IVFers. My advice: Don't take on extra work, toss dinner parties, wallpaper the powder room. Surely such projects can wait. And don't feel bad about spending a lazy Saturday afternoon in bed—you've earned it. The important thing is to maintain as much calm as possible. To do so, indulge in the things you love. Invite your partner to help out around the house by fixing dinner, scrubbing the bathroom, whatever. Let him pamper you, but don't forget to pamper him as well. Leonard, a 29-year-old graduate student, told me: "My wife's a trooper. During IVF, she barely missed a beat. Meanwhile, I sometimes got teary. I hated that she had to go through this. Plus all that uncertainty took it's toll." True, we women are usually on the frontline during IVF, but don't neglect the man in your life. Could be he's overwhelmed, too.

I'm Worried About the Possibility of Ovarian Hyperstimulation Syndrome. Can You Go Over the Symptoms?

In the previous section I mentioned that superovulatory drugs can lead to some unpleasant side effects. These include bloating, nausea, diarrhea, thirst, moodiness, and minor weight gain. Although such symptoms are not cause for major alarm, they're sometimes a precursor to ovarian hyperstimulation syndrome (OHSS). For that reason, it's essential to mention them to your RE so he or she can closely monitor you for this serious condition. Additionally, *be sure to contact your doctor immediately* if you experience any of following:

- extreme bloating and fullness above the belly button

- vomiting and/or serious diarrhea

- extreme thirst

- shortness of breath

- dark, scant, or no urine

- calf and chest pain

- weight gain of 20 pounds or more over the course of treatment, or 5 pounds in 24 hours

IVFers with one or more of these symptoms are at risk of crossing over into the danger zone—a full-fledged case of OHSS. Although relatively rare, OHSS is perhaps the single greatest risk associated with in vitro, a complication faced by about 1 to 2 percent of all patients. Severe cases can result in the leakage of hormones and fluid from the ovaries into the abdominal cavity and chest. In its worst form, OHSS can lead to blood clots, twisted ovaries, and kidney and liver damage or failure. Ironically, the patients most at risk for getting it are the ones who respond *too well* to treatment, including young women with bountiful eggs or those with polycystic ovaries. In fact, research shows that IVFers who grow 30 or more follicles and/or have estradiol readings of 6,000 picograms per milliliter have about an 80 percent chance of developing some degree of OHSS. That is, unless steps are taken to stop the condition in its tracks.

The good news is that doctors go to great lengths to carefully monitor both estrogen (via blood test) and follicle growth (via ultrasounds) to check for the red flags. If they see them, they intervene. In the past, the only way of avoiding severe OHSS was to withhold the HCG shot, then terminate the cycle. Why? Because the condition doesn't generally occur until after HCG-induced ovulation and egg retrieval, and usually gets worse if a pregnancy is achieved. That's because following egg retrieval, the aspirated follicles often fill up with fluid, causing the ovaries to swell. The symptoms of OHSS are thought to come from this fluid, which "weeps" into the abdomen, triggering extreme bloating, dangerous dehydration, and sometimes breathing difficulty. Canceling the cycle means ovulation and pregnancy can't happen, which, in most cases, causes the symptoms to gradually subside.

While that course of action helps safeguard the health of IVFers—always a priority!—it also sends them back to square one. For that reason, a number of REs have recently adopted two new treatment options. The first is to retrieve and fertilize the eggs right away, then cryopreserve the resulting embryos to use down the road in a frozen cycle—in other words, when a woman's estradiol level is no longer dangerously elevated. The second is for the IVFer to undergo a process known as "prolonged coasting." In this scenario, Lupron is continued but superovulatory meds are halted. Meanwhile, the eggs are allowed to mature slowly on their own, under the watchful eye of the RE. Three to five days later, when estradiol readings have dropped to a safe level, the HCG shot *is* given. Then, that patient proceeds to egg retrieval and beyond. While the odds of achieving a pregnancy are reduced with either intervention, both have resulted in the births of many babies.

How Do REs Track Egg Development?

Let me give you a bit of perspective. Ovaries are about the size and shape of large almonds. That's pretty small. Nevertheless, they play a crucial role in conception, for they store hundreds of thousands of eggs. These eggs are invisible to the naked eye, each housed in a tiny, blisterlike pouch called a *follicle*. During IVF, REs use a combination of Lupron (or Antagon or Centrotide) and superovulatory drugs to stimulate a large number of these eggs to mature. Doctors then face the challenge of harvesting these sand-size cells—buried deep in a woman's body—*just before* their peak of maturity. Sound challenging? It is. Fortunately, REs have two important diagnostic tools to help them track egg development and determine the optimal time frame to perform a retrieval.

The first is ultrasound. For this test, the patient lies on her back with her feet in stirrups as the RE gently inserts a probe into her vagina. Good news: It doesn't hurt, is perfectly safe, and takes a mere five minutes! How does it work? The short answer is that high-frequency sound waves are transformed into black-and-white images of the internal organs, which appear on a TV-like monitor. This monitor enables REs to not only see the ovaries, but to count and measure the enlarged follicles that reside there. An enlarged follicle usually means that an egg is ripening inside it! As the superovulatory drugs do their job, those follicles get bigger and bigger—most growing at a rate of one to two millimeters a day. Doctors keep close tabs on them with an eye toward harvesting the eggs inside *just before* they reach maturity. When is the time just right? A totally mature follicle has a diameter of about 18 to 23 millimeters. Thus, if a patient has about 10 follicles—the largest being 18 millimeters—REs can extrapolate that most of her eggs are almost full size, which means egg retrieval should happen soon.

But doctors also rely on a second diagnostic tool to make that judgment—estradiol blood tests. (To refresh your memory, estradiol is an estrogenic hormone produced by growing follicles.) First, the nurse does a simple stick in the arm and draws a vial of blood. Next, the blood is sent to the lab and tested to determine its estradiol content. Here's why: As each follicle grows, it produces more and more estradiol. Because estradiol levels are based on the quantity of eggs that are developing, each woman's reading will vary. Those with more eggs will have higher numbers and those with fewer eggs will have lower numbers. That's fine. The important thing is for the numbers to *steadily increase* throughout the stimulation phase. When that estradiol level hits a certain point (approximately 150 to 400 picograms per milliliter per mature follicle), it provides a cue—just as egg size does—that retrieval should happen *soon*.

Fertility Fact: Ovaries are the size and shape of large almonds.

These days, all REs worth their salt rely on ultrasounds *in conjunction* with estradiol readings to adjust medication dosages and pinpoint the perfect time to administer the HCG shot and retrieve eggs. Though not essential, you might consider asking your RE to share your personal levels with you. After all, the more you know, the more empowered you'll be.

Do Cycles Ever Get Canceled? Is a
Cold or Flu Something to Worry About?

Although the vast majority of cycles go smoothly, about 15 percent get canceled prior to egg retrieval. The following pie chart shows why.

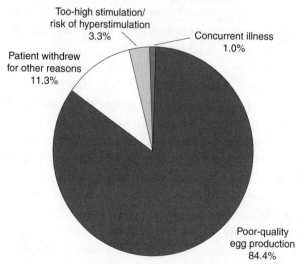

Reasons IVF Cycles Get Cancelled
From the CDC ART Report, 2001

Too-high stimulation/
risk of hyperstimulation
3.3%

Concurrent illness
1.0%

Patient withdrew
for other reasons
11.3%

Poor-quality
egg production
84.4%

As you can see, most cancellations—nearly 85 percent—happen because the patient fails to develop enough eggs. As a general rule of thumb, if three or fewer follicles grow, the IVF cycle is abandoned before the patient moves to egg retrieval. Why? Because the odds of achieving a pregnancy with three eggs or less is considered too slim to merit continuing. (Nonetheless, each case is evaluated individually and some IVFers with just an egg or two have been known to proceed with positive outcomes.) Other reasons for cancellations include a change of heart on the IVFer's part, the risk of developing ovarian hyperstimulation syndrome, or the onset of a serious illness.

Note my use of the word *serious*. Colds, low-grade flus, and the like won't derail a cycle. In fact, many a woman has slogged through in vitro while sick—myself included. During my last cycle, I came down with a nasty bug featuring a runny noise, bloodshot eyes, hacking cough, sore throat, and sallow complexion. You get the picture. I was a mess, not to mention pretty worried. But my RE shrugged off my symptoms, saying my cycle would proceed exactly as planned. Fact: Garden-variety sicknesses may make you feel crappy, but won't lead to cancellation or affect the outcome of a cycle. What will? Major health issues such as appendicitis, severe food poisoning, or an illness that elevates an IVFer's body temperature beyond 101 degrees. The latter because a high fever can have a deleterious effect on egg quality. The good news is that such temperatures are a rarity among adults so you need not be overly concerned. Nonetheless, be sure to report any illness, large or small, to your RE so he or she can advise you on the best way to treat it. (Remember, all medications, even ibuprofen, are forbidden without your doctor's say-so.)

No two ways about it, cancellations are a supreme letdown. Judith, a 31-year-old dentist, recalled her disappointment: "During my second cycle of IVF, cysts formed on my ovaries and my RE decided to cancel my cycle because the odds of my making healthy eggs were slim to none. Although she told me I could try again in a couple months, I was crushed. It seemed unfair. All that planning and effort and I barely got out of the starting gate. What a drag." A drag indeed, but not reason to throw in the towel. Many patients, including several I interviewed for this book, have bounced back from canceled cycles to try again. And I'm happy to report that a number of them, including Judith, are now proud IVF parents.

Additionally, a canceled cycle doesn't necessarily mean you won't achieve a pregnancy that month. Here's why: If a woman develops three or fewer follicles, REs will many times "convert" the IVF cycle to an intrauterine insemination (IUI) cycle. The HCG shot is still given to release the woman's eggs from her ovaries. But instead of harvesting them, the partner's sperm is injected into the uterus for possible fertilization in the fallopian tubes. True, IUI won't work for couples with tubal issues or severe male factor, and the odds aren't as good as IVF. Still, the procedure is easy, surgery free, and very low cost. As a result, it frequently makes sense to give it a try. Just ask Shawna. This 33-year-old curriculum developer recalls: "When I did IVF, only two follicles grew so my RE suggested we try IUI. I was disappointed but figured, why not? Well, the planets must have been properly aligned that day, because I got pregnant with twins. You never know!"

You never do know. If your first stab at IVF ends in a cancellation, don't give up. Speak to your RE and find out whether it makes sense to try again. In many, many cases it does. While one would be hard-pressed to say that canceled cycles are a positive thing, they often provide essential clues to your RE that can substantially improve the results in future attempts.

Commonly Asked Questions About Step 2: Retrieving Eggs

Egg retrieval, the process of harvesting ripe eggs from the ovaries, is one of the most exciting steps in the in-vitro process. Here are some answers to the big questions associated with this phase of treatment.

Can You Explain How the HCG Shot Works?

When an IVFer's eggs are almost fully developed, an injection of human chorionic gonadotropin (HCG for short) is ordered. Taking this shot is like pushing a button to trigger the final maturation of your eggs and set the stage for retrieval. If this critical step is skipped, the eggs will not be sufficiently "loosened" from the follicles that house them to enable collection. If the injection is given too early, the eggs will be premature. And if it's given too late, they'll be overly mature. It's an understatement to say timing is everything. Therefore, REs closely scrutinize each IVFer's ultrasounds and estradiol readings to pinpoint the perfect window of opportunity for administering the shot: when the majority of a patient's follicles measure between 15 and 18 millimeters in diameter and her estradiol reading closes in on 200 picograms per milliliter per follicle. The reason? Doctors know that fully mature follicles measure about 18 to 23 millimeters and have estradiol readings of 200 plus units each. Thus, a woman with 12 eggs would be ready for the HCG shot when her largest follicles reach about 18 millimeters and her estradiol reading approaches 2,400 pg/ml (2,400 ÷ 12 = 200). Will all of her eggs be strong candidates for fertilization? Probably not. A few may be immature or too mature. Still, if all goes well, a woman with 12 eggs might expect 8 or 9 to be in the "just-right" range.

Now, a word about the medication. Like many fertility-related drugs, most HCG is derived from purified urine. This time, however, it's the urine of pregnant women. Why? Pregnant women produce vast amounts of the hormone HCG, which is similar in structure to luteinizing hormone—that all-important hormone that triggers monthly ovulation. When the shot's given, the follicles containing eggs will bulge out of the ovaries and ovulation will occur in about 40 hours. REs are acutely aware of this timetable. Thus, they carefully schedule retrievals for about 36 hours following the all-important injection. That way, they'll beat ovulation *and* be able to gather the eggs near their peak of ripeness.

To accommodate this critical schedule, IVFers are often required to administer their HCG injections in the wee small hours. For example, I was told to take mine at exactly 1:30 A.M. on a Thursday. Then, my retrieval was scheduled on Saturday at 1:30 P.M. Do the math and you'll find that's exactly 36 hours later. When it comes to HCG, there isn't much wiggle room. Therefore, it is essential to be absolutely, positively precise about timing.

Fertility Fact: Although they are a great deal smaller, human eggs are similar in structure to chicken eggs.

How is the shot administered? Most types of HCG are injected intramuscularly, usually into a butt cheek in a dartlike manner. Think of the spot where the upper-outer rivet on a Levi's pocket would be. Although some women can contort their bodies to perform the shot solo, most rely on their partners to do the honors. Yes, the needle is long, but its bark is much worse than its bite. It hurts a little, but the discomfort lasts mere seconds. Theresa, a 40-year-old piano instructor, shared her big moment: "It was late at night and my boyfriend was a little nervous, but the shot went fine. It was even kind of momentous. I remember we talked about how that little syringe of HCG was like a key opening the door to our dream of a baby. Since my doctor didn't want us to drink, we toasted the occasion with wine glasses filled up with ginger ale!"

What Do I Need to Know About Egg Retrieval?

During rain or sleet or snow or hail, your RE—or another doctor at your practice—will be on hand to harvest your eggs at their pinnacle of ripeness. Nicole Noyes, an RE at New York University Program for IVF in New York City, told me, "Even on 9/11, when the city of Manhattan was in utter chaos, we managed to do every egg retrieval on time." As a New Yorker, that statement touched me. Just as there were police, firefighters, and regular folks performing heroic acts to preserve life, so, too were the IVF doctors on duty that historic day.

Egg retrievals are usually performed in an operating room–like setting, either in a hospital or at your IVF center. Although routine, it's important to understand that retrievals are surgical procedures. For that reason, patients are required not to eat or drink anything after midnight the night before as well as to bring an escort (a partner or a friend) to drive them home. In addition, they're usually given a short course of antibiotics to safeguard against the remote chance of infection, as well as Medrol, an oral steroid that helps set the stage for successful implantation.

If you're a person who hates the idea of surgery, let me set your mind at ease. Egg retrievals are safe and short, usually taking thirty minutes or less. As a result, only mild intravenous sedation is required. An IVFer dons a hospital gown and an IV is hooked up to her arm. Then before she can utter, *Does this stuff really work?*—she's out. As she sleeps, an ultrasound probe is inserted in her vagina. This enables REs to view the mature follicles, which show up as black dots on a TV-like monitor. Then, a needle is inserted into every bubblelike sack and each egg is gently sucked out into a waiting test tube. After all the mature follicles have been aspirated, the test tubes are handed off to a staff embryologist, who uses a serious microscope to hunt for eggs. Once located, the teeny eggs are removed and placed in special culture dishes—hence the term "in vitro." These dishes are filled with a nutrient-rich fluid designed to mimic the environment of the fallopian tubes. These are the magical "bedrooms" where fertilization occurs!

Now, back to the IVFer. Minutes after the process is complete, she's awakened. Yes, there's a bit of grogginess, but seldom pain or nausea. In fact, some women report a feeling akin to euphoria. After a half-hour of rest, it's time to get dressed. By then the RE can usually provide a rough count of how many eggs the embryologist has located. Stella, a 29-year-old stained-glass artisan, recounted her experience: "I remember feeling mellow and really good after my retrieval. I just lay there thinking happy thoughts. Then my RE came out and told me she'd gotten 11 eggs. It was a good day!" Following the retrieval, IVFers are sent home to take it easy for the reminder of the day. A little spotting is to be expected, but serious bleeding, cramping, or pain (all rarities) should be immediately reported to REs.

How Many Eggs Are Usually Retrieved?

Here's a small answer to that big question: Five to 12 eggs is an average yield, although some women make fewer (4 or 5) and some women make more (15 to 30 or more). As a general rule of thumb, younger women with low FSH and those with polycystic ovaries tend to produce the highest number of eggs. In fact, a few have even been known to pop as many as 50! But I wouldn't necessarily envy them. Extreme stimulation can trigger ovarian hyperstimulation syndrome and, at the very least, cause some uncomfortable side effects. Plus, when it comes to eggs, quality is much more important than quantity. One excellent egg will beat out 50 poor eggs any day of the week. Fact: Many, many an IVFer has achieved a healthy pregnancy with a very small harvest.

What Does My Partner Need to Know About Providing a Sperm Sample?

Except in cases in which a sperm donor is employed, sperm samples get collected on the day of egg retrieval. This helps to ensure they're as fresh as possible. That means, as you're undergoing the retrieval procedure, your partner will be sent to the antiseptic room to make his contribution to the cause. Some men find masturbation on demand a breeze, while others consider it a challenge on par with dancing a tango as a rhino charges. Small wonder. There's so much at stake, there's so much distraction, that performing on cue may seem like an impossibility. Still, given time and a little assistance in the form of visuals, the vast majority of men manage the task fine. Just ask Gerard. This 38-year-old insurance salesman recalls: "My wife and I did IVF two times. The first time I had to give a sperm sample, I was sent to this room that had a stack of ancient sex videos. It was like they were from the Stone Age, so things took awhile—quite a while. The second time around, I came prepared. In a brown paper bag, I brought my favorite tape and a preselected issue of *Playboy*. All I can say is that my little kit worked like a charm."

Snickers aside, Gerard's solution makes a lot of sense. Getting a fresh sample is critical to a cycle's success. So it's wise to do everything in your power to make your partner's "fifteen minutes" go well. That might mean encouraging him to bring his own visual aids or simply discussing the event to make sure he's not feeling overwhelmed. (If your mate suffers from erectile dysfunction, speak to your RE about options. Vibrators and Viagra can sometimes help.)

In addition, encourage your partner to heed your RE's instructions to the letter. He'll likely be asked to refrain from sexual activity for one to three days prior (but not more!), take a short course of antibiotics, and vigorously wash his hands before the deed. No kidding, even a little bacteria can put the kibosh on an otherwise promising sample. Make certain, too, that your partner has some frozen sperm banked just in case. Cryopreserved sperm has been known to save cycles when a fresh sample gets contaminated or your mate comes down with a serious illness. High temperatures can seriously compromise both the quality and quantity of sperm.

Finally, Gerard advises men to take the experience in stride: "Producing a sample for IVF is definitely a little surreal so it's probably best to relax and just go with the weirdness. I remember putting my semen in this little two-sided cabinet for pick up. I thought, there goes the jar that may contain half the genetic makeup of my child. And it did. My son Ian is almost two."

What If My Partner Needs to Have His Sperm Extracted? Does It Hurt?

Some men have no sperm in their ejaculate at all. In many cases that's due to blocked or missing ejaculatory ducts. Either way, just because sperm isn't present in a sperm sample doesn't mean it's nonexistent. Often, healthy sperm are alive and well in the *epididymis* (the duct leading out of the testes where the sperm matures) or the testicles themselves. The only challenge is extracting them. For previous generations, that was a major stumbling block—a task formerly on par with removing a million bucks from a combinationless safe. Today, however, it's possible for millions of men to have biological children thanks to a new breed of sperm retrieval methods used with IVF. Two of the major processes include:

❧ **Micro Epididymal Sperm Aspiration (MESA):** Some men have blocked or absent ejaculatory ducts—either due to vasectomy or a congenital defect. In this procedure sperm are carefully aspirated from the epididymis.

❧ **Testicular Sperm Extraction (TESE):** For men with a missing or damaged epididymis, it is now possible to remove sperm directly from the manufacturer—the testicles. In this process, small samples of testicular tissue are obtained by needle biopsy. Then, a few sperm are painstakingly removed from it.

If you think your partner will require one of these procedures, speak to your RE. Chances are he or she can recommend an experienced urologist well versed in sperm extraction and accustomed to working with in vitro clinics. The price tag? TESE costs in the neighborhood of $1,000, while the more expensive MESA costs about $2,500. (Not cheap, but not off the charts in the context of IVF.) Both microsurgeries require only a few hours of time and men can return to their normal routines right away. They're also safe and, thanks to local anesthesia, nearly pain free. And here's more good news: When used in conjunction with ICSI, fertilization rates with testicular sperm extraction are no different from rates with ejaculated sperm. Maura, a 31-year-old administrative assistant, shared how she and her husband dealt with this situation: "When I couldn't get pregnant, I assumed it was me. Then we did all this testing and found out my husband, Jed, had sperm in his testicles, but not in his semen. When the doctor mentioned TESE, Jed's face went white. I could tell he was squeamish. Still, he wanted kids as much as I did so he bit the bullet and did it without complaint. To say thanks, I made his favorite 'manly meal'—steak and potatoes. He really earned it." If your partner requires sperm extraction, try to give him a little extra TLC. Even if he doesn't show it, chances are he needs your love and support, just as much as you need his.

Commonly Asked Questions About Step 3: Developing Embryos

Embryo development happens behind the scenes—in an off-limits laboratory room. For that reason, this step is perhaps the least understood. Here, you'll find information to help shed light on the amazing process of fertilization.

Can You Tell Me a Little About the IVF Lab?

IVF labs aren't pretty places. If you ever have the privilege of visiting one, you won't find mahogany desks and plush carpeting. Rather, you'll see a spartan workspace filled with lots of high-tech equipment, including incubators, fancy microscopes, and an assortment of complex micromanipulation tools. Plus a whole lot of stainless steel. In this sealed world, a customized air filter hums to limit dust particles and admittance is by invitation only. It is the domain of scrub-clad embryologists—a unique breed of doctors who eat, drink, and sleep embryo development.

It is the place where freshly retrieved eggs and sperm are delivered to meet and mate.

The window of opportunity for fertilization is small: It must take place within a few hours of harvest. Fortunately, good embryologists have this make-or-break step of IVF down to a science. First, the fragile eggs are gently washed, graded for their maturity, and transferred to individual culture dishes filled with nutrient-rich fluid. As the eggs rest, the semen sample is meticulously "processed" to remove debris and obtain the greatest concentration of strong, healthy, motile sperm. This involves spinning the semen in a machine called a *centrifuge*, which separates out the sperm and removes proteins and enzymes from their heads—a process that readies them to penetrate the egg. Next, unless ICSI is being employed, 50,000 to 100,000 of the finest specimens are added in with each egg. The culture dishes are then placed in a customized incubator maintained at a woman's body temperature. Despite the absence of candlelight and romantic music, it is here that the most primitive form of the mating ritual takes place. If all goes well, a single sperm will burrow through the shell of the egg—nearly 600 times its size—to fertilize it.

About 18 hours after insemination, embryologists open the incubator and check for the first tentative signs of fertilization: the formation of two clear bubbles on the egg called *the pronuclei*. One represents the genetic contribution of the male and the other represents the contribution of the female. When these two bubbles fuse, a new life may be formed. But embryologists know not to get overly excited at this stage.

The bad news is that a number of these very early embryos won't make it, petering out along the way because of invisible chromosomal damage or other problems related to egg and/or sperm quality. The good news is a lot of them *do* make it! About 60 to 80 percent will continue the amazing process of cell division. Within 48 hours, promising embryos contain two or more cells and, within 72 hours, they contain six to eight. If cells are left to divide and redivide for five days—to the blastocyst stage—embryos will have an impressive 64 to 100 cells!

Fertility Fact: Some degree of fragmentation is found in about 80 percent of IVF embryos.

Human fertilization is a remarkable process, even to seasoned embryologists. Hence, they take their role very seriously—carefully evaluating each embryo by noting its number of cells, cell symmetry, and degree of fragmentation (minuscule bits of the cytoplasm that form beadlike blobs on the cells—kind of like pills on an old sweater). Embryos with numerous, equally sized spherical cells and minimal fragmentation have the best shot at thriving. But embryologists have a few tricks up their sleeves to help eggs, sperm, and embryos in need. One is called *rescue ICSI*. In this procedure, eggs that fail to become fertilized by the sperm placed in their lab dishes are injected with individual sperm in an attempt to "rescue" their chances of becoming embryos. (See page 243 for more.) Another strategy is assisted hatching—often a key part of the protocol for women 37 and beyond. Why? The embryos of older IVFers tend to have thicker shells, which reduce the odds of successful implantation. To nip this problem in the bud, a tiny hole is "drilled" in the shell of the embryo (either chemically or with a laser), thereby enabling it to hatch out of the shell and attach itself to the uterine lining. Occasionally, doctors even go to the extreme length of performing a process called *fragmentation removal,* in which they painstakingly remove the beadlike cell fragments in an effort to "clean up" the embryo and streamline cell division.

I think you get the picture. Embryologists carefully monitor and nurture each tiny charge. In fact, in many ways, the in-vitro lab is like a hospital nursery. No, there aren't any cooing infants in pink- and blue-striped caps, but there *is* the potential for them. Thanks, in great part, to these behind-the-scenes doctors with a passion for small things.

My RE Thinks We'll Need Intracytoplasmic Sperm Injection. Can You Explain the Process?

If you've been reading this book straight through, you've surely come across countless mentions of the futuristic-sounding *intracytoplasmic sperm injection,* acronym ISCI. That's because it's a subject close to my heart. Had this technology not been developed in the early nineties, my husband and I would probably not have been able to be biological parents. Nor would thousands of other IVFers facing the roadblock of male factor. Before that, there was no consistently effective way to address the problem of poor-quality sperm—that is, sperm incapable of fertilizing eggs on their own.

How does ICSI work? Step one, the egg is held in place with a narrow tube called a *pipette.* Step two, the needle is used to immobilize and pick up a single sperm. Step three, a needle is positioned inside the pipette and the sperm is injected through the egg's shell directly into the cytoplasm, where, if all goes well, fertilization will soon occur. Sound amazing? It is. Especially when you consider the scale: An egg is about the size of a grain of sand and a sperm is many, many times smaller. For that reason, embryologists must perform this fertilization feat while peering through the lenses of a high-powered microscope. Artists specializing in intricate paintings on the heads of pins have nothing on them!

At its inception, ICSI was only employed in cases of extreme male factor. Today, however, the technique is used in nearly 50 percent of all IVF cycles, including those in which seemingly normal sperms fail to fertilize the eggs they are paired with. The latter process is called *rescue ICSI.* Additionally, a few doctors have decided to *always* do ICSI, regardless of sperm quality. "We're implementing a 100 percent

ICSI," reports Dr. Geoffrey Sher, founder of the Sher Institute for Reproductive Medicine in Las Vegas, Nevada. The reasoning? Like a head start in a race, they believe that "short-cutting" the fertilization process can't help but boost success rates. But others REs beg to differ, countering that adding a single drop of sperm to lab dishes can do the job just fine and is far less expensive. How much are we talking here? The price of ICSI can tack $750 to $2,500 onto the price of a cycle. Still, for many that's a small price to pay for the chance for a biological baby—or in my case, two!

Fertility Fact: The first "ICSI baby" was born in Australia in 1986.

I Understand Embryos Are Graded. Can You Explain the Process?

The idea of getting grades during the course of a cycle may not sit well with some readers. As a less-than-stellar student, I cringe at the mere mention of anything that smacks of report cards. The fact of the matter is, however, that the grading process is a key step in the IVF process. Why? It helps REs choose the very best embryos to transfer to the uterus, which vastly improves pregnancy rates.

In the future, the in-vitro community will likely adopt a uniform grading system. In the meantime, any quality IVF center has developed its own. Some favor letter grades (A, B, C, D, E); some favor number grades (1, 2, 3, 4, 5); and some favor percentages (100, 90, 80, etc.). Whatever the method, the intent is the same: to carefully assess each embryo with an eye toward selecting the healthiest specimens for transfer. Embryos are evaluated in three major categories:

- **Cell number:** The more cells the better!

- **Cell regularity:** Even, spherical cells are a good thing.

- **Degree of fragmentation:** The less *fragmentation*—little bits of the cytoplasm that "bud off" and form tiny blobs on the cells—the better.

As a general rule, embryos that receive the highest marks in these areas stand the highest chance of resulting in a healthy pregnancy. However, there are no guarantees. Exquisite-looking, A+ embryos sometimes fail to implant, just as homely, C- embryos occasionally do. Now, you're probably wondering if there's a correlation between perfect embryos and perfect kids. True, low-quality embryos are far less likely than high-quality embryos to become babies. But if they do, rest assured that they'll be just as cute, strong, brilliant, talented, and *perfect* as any other kid on the block. Dr. Jeffrey Boldt, an experienced embryologist at the Southeastern Center for Fertility and Reproductive Surgery in Knoxville, Tennessee, agrees: "Yes, ugly embryos are walking around as beautiful children!"

Now, a word about what accounts for inferior embryos. While some mystery still remains, the leading causes are poor-quality eggs, poor-quality sperm, inadequate stimulation, and inferior lab conditions. Just as it's a good idea to get a sense of your ballpark chances of succeeding with IVF, it's a good idea to get a gauge on the state of your embryos. Therefore, it's probably wise to ask your RE to share info about the evaluation of your "little ones" (as well as the finer points of the scoring system employed). In my opinion, dealing with the facts is always the best course of action.

What's a Blastocyst?

When it comes to IVF, the term *blastocyst* gets bandied about a lot. I have to admit it used to throw me. It's one of those scientific words—like *phylum* or *antigen*—that's somehow intimidating. So let me define it here: A blastocyst is an advanced embryo that has divided and divided and divided until it has 64 to 100 cells. Blastocyst embryos are mature and nearly ready to implant in the uterine lining. They contain an inner mass of cells destined to become the fetus *and* an outer layer of cells destined to become the placenta. If a brand-new embryo is a freshman, a blastocyst embryo is a senior. Blastocysts don't happen overnight—it takes about five days to get there (with many an embryo dying out before reaching this critical state). That being said, if an embryo *does* reach the blastocyst stage, it stands a pretty good chance of thriving in utero and developing into a fetus.

For that reason, most quality IVF practices make it their business to perform a number of transfers with blastocysts—or *five days after* embryo retrieval as opposed to three.

This wasn't always the case. In the early days of IVF, almost all transfers were performed three days after retrieval. That worked pretty well, but it was often hard to choose the best embryos to transfer. After all, early embryos of six to eight cells look pretty similar. Like marathoners at the 10-mile mark, it's sometimes hard to tell which of those embryos have the right stuff to go the distance. That got REs thinking and some began experimenting with delaying transfer dates. Bingo! The strategy seemed to be working—pregnancy rates were subtly improving. Long story short: In the late 1990s, "day-five blastocyst transfers" started gaining momentum. The reason? They enable embryologists and REs to better determine which embryos are the strongest candidates for transfer. Let's say, for example, a couple has 10 thriving embryos. On day 3 it might not be too clear which ones are the cream of the crop. If, however, those embryos are allowed to develop to the blastocyst stage, the frontrunners—those with the most cells and most symmetrical structure—will be far more apparent. Then, REs can select the heartiest-appearing two or three for transfer and freeze the other contenders for future cycles.

But blastocyst transfers aren't right for everyone. When a couple has a smaller number of thriving embryos—say two or three—performing a day 3 transfer with embryos at the six- to eight-cell stage probably makes more sense. Here's the reason: If *all* of the good embryos are going to be transferred anyway, then comparing them at a later stage is a moot point. Plus, many REs believe that embryos stand a better chance of surviving in utero than in a lab dish. For that reason, women who are not candidates for blastocyst transfers shouldn't feel disappointed. Fact: The vast majority of IVF babies are the result of day-three transfers, my own included. With a total of six embryos—three rated "excellent" and three rated "poor"—it was pretty apparent the best option for me was to transfer the three excellent ones three days after my retrieval. Well, two implanted and I have my precious twins. The moral of my story: While day-five blastocyst transfers result in slightly higher pregnancy rates, day-three transfers tend to work very well, too!

Commonly Asked Questions
About Step 4: Transferring Embryos

Embryo transfer is an exhilarating and stressful step. Eggs have been successfully fertilized, but will these develop into healthy fetuses? This section addresses the many issues IVFers face at this juncture, including the all-important question of how many embryos to transfer.

How Many Embryos Should We Transfer?
Ahhh, the million-dollar question. To reduce the risk of multiple births, many countries have adopted national policies regarding embryo transfer. In England, doctors are allowed to transfer a max of three and, in Scandinavia, most clinics limit IVFers to one. At present, there are no such laws in the United States, but there are definitely trends. Let's take a look at a relevant pie graph.

Number of Embryos
Transferred During IVF
From the CDC ART Report, 2001

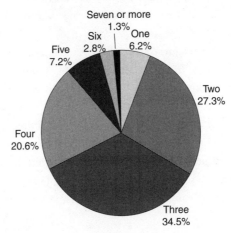

Seven or more
1.3%
Six 2.8%
One 6.2%
Five 7.2%
Two 27.3%
Four 20.6%
Three 34.5%

* Total does not equal 100% due to rounding.

As you can see, the vast majority of IVFers—nearly 89 percent—receive between one and four embryos. Now, let me say a word about the

11 percent who receive five, seven, or more. These days, REs will only transfer such large quantities if they are convinced, without a shadow of a doubt, that the embryo quality is so low that no more than two will implant. And they are the exceptions to the rule. The vast majority of clinics have semirigid policies regarding the number of embryos REs are allowed to transfer. As a general rule, most limit patients under 37 to one to three embryos and patients over 37 to one to four. That's because, like their European colleagues, American doctors worry about the risk of multiples. At present, 32 percent of patients who achieve pregnancies have twins and nearly 4 percent have triplets or more.

While it might sound appealing to bounce a bunch of babies on your knee, the reality is that it's a major challenge. Multiple gestation poses some very serious health risks to mother and babies—including preeclampsia and birth defects—that become increasingly more pronounced with each additional fetus. Fact: In nearly 40 percent of triplet and quads pregnancies, at least one of the infants suffers from a physical and/or neurological complication related to premature delivery. Multiples can also lead to major financial and child-rearing problems. While one or two newborns can be manageable, three or four demanding babies can test the resolve and resources of even the sturdiest parents.

For these reasons and more, it's wise to have a serious conversation with your RE about transfer options. Chances are, he or she will have strong, almost ironclad opinions on the topic. Still, there may well be room for a little negotiation. Does that mean you can get six "excellent" embryos transferred? Unless your RE is a quack—no way! However, you might be able to make a case for getting four "good" embryos implanted as opposed to three, provided you're willing to face the possibility of multiples. The point is that every IVFer's transfer must be *carefully* thought through. Here are the primary factors to consider:

❧ **Your embryo quality:** The better the embryo, the more likely it is to implant and become a fetus.

❧ **Your comfort level with risky pregnancies and multiples:** If embryo quality is good, two or three embryos could well result in two or three fetuses. That will make your pregnancy and parenting more challenging.

❧ **Your comfort level with selective reduction:** Selective reduction is a widely practiced medical procedure in which couples elect to terminate an early fetus at the 11th or 12th week of pregnancy to help safeguard the health of the other fetus or fetuses. In this outpatient procedure, a sonogram is performed, then a needle containing a special chemical—usually potassium chloride—is injected into the fetus. (Doctors do several tests in an attempt to select the one that is already the most at risk.) The heart is stopped and the fetus is usually reabsorbed into the tissue of the uterus without pain or significant bleeding. The process is safe, although complications do occur in roughly 2 to 5 percent of cases (including the loss of the other fetuses).

Without a doubt, selective reduction is one of the most difficult aspects of in vitro fertilization. Sure, it's tempting for couples to bury their heads in the sand and not decide their stance on this difficult issue. But frankly, that's just not an option. In vitro requires that we search our souls and make tough personal choices. As a result, many readers of this book will come to terms with the possible need for selective reduction to reduce quads to triplets, triplets to twins, and even twins to singletons. While others, for religious or ethical reasons, will find the concept outside of their comfort zone. June, a 32-year-old teacher trainer, shared her experience with me: "I elected to have three embryos transferred. Then I learned I was pregnant with triplets. At first, I was elated to be pregnant with three, then it sunk in: How would we be able to care for and afford them? Plus, I worried about the toll a high-risk pregnancy could take on the babies, especially if the triplets arrived several weeks early. After much discussion, my husband and I decided to do selective reduction. Although the procedure was pretty straightforward, it was kind of hard. Still, I look at my beautiful twins, now four, and I know we made the right choice." Diane, a 40-year-old pharmacist, came to a different conclusion: "We thought and thought about it, but I just could not get comfortable with the idea of the selective reduction procedure. As a result, we decided to play it safe and transfer only two embryos to guarantee that we didn't have more than twins."

Are you prepared to deal with the risk of multiples? Is selective reduction something you would or wouldn't consider? These important questions should be explored before or early in your cycle to help determine exactly how many embryos to transfer. Even one extra can make a difference! Listen to your RE. He or she likely has sound opinions (not to mention vetoing power). Listen to your partner. You're in this together. Listen to your heart. It will help you decide what's best for you.

How Can We Be Assured That We Get **Our** *Embryos?*

You've probably seen a sensational news story that goes something like this: Nice couple undergoes in vitro, brings home an adorable baby, then comes to discover the baby is the biological offspring of another nice couple. Tempers flair, a nasty trial ensues, and everyone's miserable. Cringing at the thought? If so, let me offer some words of comfort. First, lab mix-ups are extremely rare. In the whole history of IVF, there have been only a few. Second, all reputable centers have devised elaborate systems of checks and cross-checks to ensure that such mistakes don't happen. For example, every test tube, lab dish, and incubator containing sperm, eggs, and embryos is *always* meticulously labeled with the patient's name and social security number. Some centers even go to the length of assigning each IVFer a distinct color, then color-coding all their "property" as well.

In addition, signatures are required whenever these items go anywhere—even across the hall—with only a handful of trusted staffers ever having access to them. Finally, during all egg retrievals and embryo transfers, the female patient wears a hospital wristband and is officially asked to state her full name loudly and clearly to make certain she's correctly identified. Emma, a 42-year-old adjunct professor, recalls: "During my embryo transfer, I was lying there with my feet in stirrups. First the RE asked me my name. Then the nurse asked my name. Then she checked my hospital bracelet, and then they both initialed some form. The odd thing was they both knew me very well!

All that official business felt a little impersonal, but, in the end, I'm glad they were so careful."

If you're worried about the potential for lab mix-ups, ask your RE to outline the security precautions they employ. Chances are their rigorous standards will cross this concern right off your list.

What Do I Need to Know About Embryo Transfer?

Just writing about embryo transfer brings back a flood of visceral emotions, including trepidation, exhilaration, and hope. The experience was momentous—right up there with my high school graduation, trek to Russia, wedding, and birth of my sons. Paradoxically, embryo transfer *is* and *isn't* a big deal. Yes, there's a lot at stake, but the process is surprisingly brief, taking little more time than a routine pap smear.

As with egg retrievals, it behooves IVFers to be absolutely punctual. Partners are an asset, but strong fragrances are not. Some REs believe that perfumes, even strong shampoos, can have a deleterious effect on fragile embryos. Here's the process in a nutshell: Step one, you don a hospital gown and lie on an examination-type table with your feet in stirrups. Step two, a speculum is inserted into your vagina and excess cervical mucus is removed. (With all the fertility drugs, some women generate a lot of it.) Step three, the RE gently glides the catheter into position. Step four, the embryos—generally two to four—are injected into your uterus. The RE then passes the catheter to an embryologist who checks it under a microscope to make sure all of the embryos have been deposited. (In rare cases, one is left behind and can be re-injected.) Time elapsed: about 10 to 15 minutes.

After the procedure, you'll continue to lie on your back for half an hour or so. To foster a positive experience, many IVF centers encourage the male partner to witness the event, even hold his wife's hand. This helps her feel supported and helps him feel connected. In many cases, too, couples are presented with microscope photos of their developing embryos to help them visualize their babies-to-be. In addition, some bring their own talismans. Here's Megan, a 27-year-old musician: "At the start of IVF my husband got me this little tan teddy bear and said, 'We'll give this to our son or daughter when our IVF adventure is over.' That teddy bear had a lot of meaning so I brought him to my transfer." As for me, I closed my eyes and imagined the tiny embryos landing on my uterine wall like minuscule sky divers. No matter that the image bore no resemblance to reality. It made me feel good.

For many, personal artifacts and visualization promote a relaxed frame of mind. However, if all else fails, a single Valium—provided by an RE—can sometimes do the trick. (Ask yours about the possibility if you think it will help.) The fact is, some women love embryo transfers, while others find them relatively stressful. Both responses are valid. If you fall into the latter camp, don't despair. Many an IVFer felt that way and ended up with a positive pregnancy test.

Will I Be Able to Feel the Embryos in My Uterus?

An embryo is a microscopic mass of cells about the size of a speck of dust. Thus, even the most sensitive, body-conscious woman will not be able to "feel" them. Janice, a 35-year-old executive recruiter, recalls: "When my embryo transfer was over and I was sent home, it was a bit of a letdown. I mean here was this momentous occasion, and aside from some nervousness, I felt totally normal. I don't know what I was expecting, but it wasn't *normal*." There's no question an embryo transfer is a milestone of sorts. But don't expect the clouds to part and a hundred angels to descend from the heavens trumpeting the arrival of your new pregnancy. The truth is pregnancies don't occur until a few days *after* a transfer. In the meantime, your embryos will float around your uterus, like little astronauts, continuing their essential cell division. Then if all goes well, one or more will touch down on a nice strip of the uterine wall, burrow in, and begin producing the hormone HCG—the first sign of pregnancy. So don't worry if you don't feel anything. Hopefully, that will all change in the months to come.

Should I Rest Up After My Transfer?

With regard to the question of resting up after a transfer, REs agree to disagree. Some are quick to order strict bed rest for a day or two, while others confidently tell their patients to resume normal activity. Here's Ruby's story, a 37-year-old retail manager: "When I asked if I should go to bed following my transfer, my RE kind of laughed. Then she told me a story about herself—how after she'd gotten pregnant naturally she went back and did the math to figure out when she conceived. Turns out it was in the middle of a ski trip in which she fell down tons and tons of times. And still, the embryo implanted. After hearing that, I decided to go to work. Getting back into my routine felt right. And yes, I ended up pregnant." Lynne, a 39-year-old computer programmer, took a different tack: "During my first cycle, I didn't rest and I didn't get pregnant. So I changed my tune for cycle number two. I laid on the couch for three full days, while my husband waited on me hand and foot. I don't know if it made a difference, but I do know I got pregnant."

Two approaches, two pregnancies. What should you do? First and foremost, follow your RE's advice. And if he or she doesn't have a strong opinion, my suggestion is to err on the side of taking it easy. Although a lot of doctors will tell you bed rest doesn't help, it certainly won't hurt. And if you lay low, you'll know that you did everything in your power to foster implantation. Plus, a couple days in bed with favorite magazines and a pint of ice cream doesn't sound too shabby now does it?

Can You Explain the Process of Freezing Embryos? What Are My Options Regarding Extras?

Here's a riddle: How is it possible for twins to be born several years apart? Answer: With the miracle of embryo freezing! If a couple with an IVF baby has frozen embryos from the same cycle, they can tap that supply at a later date. Then, if all goes according to plan, a second baby will be born who's several years younger than its fraternal twin. Sound incredible? It is. Embryo freezing—otherwise known as *cryopreservation*—got its start in 1983, the year the very first baby was born from a frozen embryo at world-famous Monash IVF in Australia. Since then, the technology has vastly improved, making the cryopreservation of embryos a wise option for many couples. To date, thousands of healthy babies have been born from so-called frozen cycles (see Chapter 10 for more information).

How does the embryo-freezing process work? At the time of an IVFer's transfer, one to four of the best embryos will be chosen to go into her uterus. In about 25 to 30 percent of cases, though, a surplus of healthy embryos remain. By healthy I mean those with a rating of good or excellent. (Most practices counsel against freezing poor-grade embryos because the chance of achieving pregnancies with them are very low.) These extra embryos can be successfully frozen following either day 3 or day 5 blastocyst transfers. They can even be frozen on day 1 at the pronuclear stage. Here's how it works: First, water in the embryos is replaced with a cryoprotectant; this acts as an antifreeze and keeps damaging ice crystals from forming. Next, the embryos are placed in thin test tubes called *straws* and slowly frozen. They are then plunged into a special storage tank filled with liquid nitrogen and cooled to a bone-numbing –196 degrees Celsius. There, they'll remain until they're tapped for subsequent cycles.

Is embryo freezing the right choice for everyone? No. There are some IVFers whose religious or personal beliefs bar them from considering cryopreservation. (These individuals can choose to donate their fresh embryos to other couples, make them available for scientific research, or let them "peter out" in the lab dish.) For many IVFers, however, freezing extra embryos makes perfect sense. Frozen embryos provide a second chance when a fresh cycle fails as well as a significant head start on another baby if it succeeds. Although success rates for frozen cycles aren't as high as for fresh cycles—about 20 percent versus 26 percent—they're far less expensive and invasive. But there are a couple more downsides. First, there's the annual cost of storage—$600 or more a year. Second, there's the responsibility. It's important to understand that storing frozen embryos requires essential follow-through on the part of couples. If annual payments aren't made in a timely manner or you lose touch with your clinic, the embryos stand the risk of being destroyed. In addition, many practices will only keep them for five years. After that, decisions have to be made whether to move them to another facility, destroy them, offer them up for scientific research, or donate them to other couples. The latter option can usually be done through your in-vitro clinic or an embryo adoption program such as Snowflakes. (See *Resources* for more information.)

When it comes to extra embryos, there are a number of critical decisions to be made. For that reason, all IVF practices require patients to read and sign serious consent forms regarding these options. My advice? Discuss the topic with your mate in a calm atmosphere to arrive at the right choice for both of you.

I've Heard It's Now Possible to Freeze Eggs. Is That True?

Yes and no. Despite a few isolated success stories—including the birth of the first "frozen-egg baby" in 1986—it's currently a very tall order to freeze and thaw eggs for use in IVF. That's largely due to their fragile, liquid-y composition, which makes cryopreservation a challenge. But strides are being made. Dr. Jeffrey Boldt, an embryologist at the Southeastern Center for Fertility and Reproductive Surgery in Knoxville, Tennessee, reports that "In the past few months we've achieved a number of pregnancies and births from frozen eggs." In addition, a biotech company called ViaCell has developed a procedure to streamline the freezing process that is currently in clinical trials. If that testing goes well, widespread egg freezing may be just around the corner.

Fertility Fact: To date, a handful of births have resulted from frozen, thawed, then fertilized eggs.

That's a pretty big deal. Consider the impact it will have on young women facing cancer treatments or those whose biological clocks are ticking, but haven't yet met Mr. Right. Soon they'll have the option of freezing healthy eggs to use down the road when the time is just right to have a baby. Who knows? Perhaps it will even become a rite of passage for women to cryopreserve a batch of eggs on their 30th birthdays—just in case.

Commonly Asked Questions About
Step 5: Preparing the Uterine Lining

The preparation of the uterine lining isn't an exciting step, but it is an essential one because it helps incoming embryos successfully implant. For that reason, IVFers are required to begin daily progesterone treatments around the time of embryo transfer. To learn more, read on.

Why Is It So Important to Prepare the Uterine Lining?

A couple can have the most beautiful embryos on the face of the planet, but if the uterine lining—also known as the *endometrium*—isn't just right, there's no hope of sustaining a pregnancy. Why? Consider the walls of the room you're in. Because they're dry, a speck of dust won't adhere. Now imagine them coated with grape jelly. Would that speck of dust adhere? Probably so. This same principle can be applied to the walls of your uterus. For an embryo to take hold, the endometrium must be thick—REs want to see at least 9 millimeters—nutrient rich, and sticky. That calls for two hormones: estrogen and progesterone.

Women's bodies produce both of them naturally. Around ovulation time, there's an influx of estrogen and, shortly thereafter, a rise in progesterone. These hormones work together to build a thick, welcoming endometrium—the perfect habitat for arriving embryos. But, while supplemental estrogen isn't generally administered during standard IVF, progesterone is. Here's why: First, some women's normal progesterone levels are simply inadequate. Second, research suggests that superovulatory drugs can reduce natural progesterone production—meaning the uterine lining won't be lush enough to promote implantation. For both reasons, almost all IVFers take progesterone supplements. Expect daily treatments to begin around the time of embryo transfer and to extend until your pregnancy test—and well beyond—if a pregnancy is achieved.

What Are Progesterone Treatments Like?

Although the majority of IVFers receive progesterone by intramuscular injection, a few practices prescribe it in the form of vaginal suppositories or a gel. The latter options spare women the—literal—pain in the butt of shots. (If you're a shot-hater, ask your RE about these alternatives.) For most, progesterone treatments are no big deal. Mine were delivered via injection, by the loving hand of my husband. Because progesterone is viscous, it took a few seconds for the thick fluid to exit the needle and enter my muscle. That caused some stinging and black-and-blue marks. But I'd take that pain over a stubbed toe any day of the week. And the bruising was my little secret. It wasn't like my derriere was going up on a gallery wall anytime soon.

Next, a word about side effects. Mine were minor. I felt kind of PMS-y, but that was it. Others don't get off quite so easily. Toni, a 39-year-old customs broker, recalls, "I found the progesterone more difficult than the superovulatory drugs. It made me feel achy and puffed up—kind of like my insides were coated with ten layers of paint." Progesterone, like other drugs on the IVF menu, has a range of annoying side effects that include bloating, nausea, stomach pain, constipation, diarrhea, headaches, breast tenderness, joint pain, drowsiness, nervousness, and the annoying need to pee in the middle of the night. In addition, the injections occasionally cause red bumps and skin rashes. Often that's due to a sensitivity to the peanut or sesame seed oil the progesterone comes packed in. Thus, if you know you're allergic to one or the other, be sure to inform your RE beforehand so he or she can adjust your prescription accordingly.

Do REs Have Other Tools to Foster Implantation?

Although the use of progesterone is de rigueur, some REs choose to supplement it with baby aspirin, heparin, nitroglycerine patches, prednisone, human chorionic gonadotropin (HCG), estrogen, even Viagra. All of these are tools thought to improve the state of the uterine lining, helping to create the optimal endometrium for successful implantation. Which are the most effective? The jury is still out. In the meantime, different doctors have different hunches—and favorites. Therefore, if you happen to be prescribed one (or more) of these medications, it's wise to ask why.

Commonly Asked Questions About
Step 6: Taking the Pregnancy Test(s)

The first pregnancy test is usually performed about 10 days to two weeks after embryo transfer. Although it amounts to no more than a simple stick in the arm to draw blood, for many it's the most nerve-racking step in the process. In the following section, you'll find information and tips to help maintain calm during the pinnacle of the roller-coaster ride.

Will I Be Able to Tell If I'm Pregnant?
Are There Ways to Keep Calm Before My Test?

There's no question that the period between embryo transfer and pregnancy test can be difficult. With the exception of daily progesterone treatments, there is nothing to do but wait and wait and obsess. I remember those days well. One particular afternoon I couldn't turn off my brain so I decided to go to a movie carefully selected for its mindlessness. On my way to the theater, I passed my favorite clothing store and noticed that a fabulous red dress was marked down to half-price. A part of me wanted to rush in and buy it, but the other part of me said, *No, if all goes well you'll soon be wearing maternity garb.* That made sense, so I kept on walking. At the theater, the ticket seller was clearly with child. *Was that a sign?* Once inside, I had a sudden urge to devour a giant tub of buttery popcorn—a choice I would have previously found, well, rather disgusting. *Could this be my first pickles-and-ice-cream type craving?* I wasn't sure, but opted for the popcorn anyway. After munching away for the better part of an hour, I developed a mild case of indigestion. *Was this further evidence that I was pregnant?* I tried to concentrate on the screen, but kept getting distracted by every nuance of my body. Suddenly, I detected a slight heaviness in my abdomen. *Oh no—did that mean my period wasn't far behind?* The mere thought caused me to burst into tears—which no doubt confounded nearby patrons. After all, this was an action adventure, not *Gone with the Wind.* As the credits rolled, I shuffled out—ashamed, emotionally drained, utterly clueless.

The moral of my little story? It's fairly impossible for even the most body-attentive IVFer to assess the state of her uterus. First, there's all that progesterone coursing through your system. Second, the onset of menstruation—namely, cramping, moodiness, changes in appetite, even spotting—is surprisingly similar to the earliest stages of pregnancy. Courtney, a 40-year-old interior decorator, remembers it this way: "After my embryo transfer, it was a roller coaster ride. One day I thought I was pregnant, the next I thought I wasn't. Then there were a few spots of brown blood. I freaked out and called my IVF center. They calmed me down, saying that's sometimes a sign of pregnancy. Turns out I *was* pregnant and the bleeding had to do with the embryo implanting in the uterine lining. Things worked out well, but that last phase of treatment was a real challenge."

I have to say that I agree with Courtney. The last phase of treatment *is* a challenge. Still, trying to maintain a regular routine can help. A positive attitude can help, too. But don't beat up on yourself for those moments you're feeling a little or a lot pessimistic. As I mentioned previously, negative emotions come with the territory and will *not* affect the outcome of your cycle. If I had a nickel for every IVFer who told me she feared she wasn't pregnant then was, I'd be a wealthy woman. My advice: Treat yourself especially well with movies, naps, books, retail therapy, country drives, baking, whatever makes you happy. Just don't bite off more than you can chew. The stress of awaiting your results may release adrenaline, which can leave you pretty tuckered out. That means it's probably not a good time to undertake big projects. It is, however, a good time to recruit family, friends, and your mate to pamper you. Courtney concurs: "Awaiting the pregnancy test kind of sucked. But it helped to have my husband catering to my every need. He even unloaded the dishwasher!"

Is There Anything I Should Do to Prepare for My Pregnancy Test?

On the eve of my second IVF pregnancy test (following a failed cycle) my husband and I ventured out to our favorite Italian restaurant. My spaghetti and meatballs remained untouched. But the dinner was pretty cathartic. I hadn't planned on saying anything, but the words tumbled out. I told him I had no idea whether or not I was pregnant. But if the pregnancy test was negative, I wanted to try in vitro again. That is, provided our RE agreed that it made sense. My husband concurred and we clicked water glasses, toasting the promise of our cycle while acknowledging the fact that it could end in failure. Was it a difficult conversation? Yes. But poking my head out of the pink cloud made me feel better prepared for whatever lay ahead. And confirming that our situation might call for even a third IVF attempt gave me courage to face my pregnancy test without feeling as if it was my last chance.

Is a similar conversation appropriate for you? Maybe not. Still, I think it makes sense to have a short conversation with your mate in which you acknowledge the possibility that IVF might not work *this time around*. While one can never be fully prepared for a negative pregnancy test, talking about it beforehand may help a little. Nevertheless, always, always remain hopeful, for the numbers are on your side! Fact: About 70 percent of all IVFers end up bringing a baby home following one to three cycles. Those are pretty good odds.

Can I Use an At-Home Pregnancy Test?

The answer is yes, with the caveat that it's probably not such a great idea. Here's the reason: Urine-based kits purchased at drugstores are not nearly as sensitive as the blood tests administered at IVF centers. That means a drugstore kit could actually *miss* the earliest signs of pregnancy and result in a false negative. Plus, it certainly won't provide an indication of whether you're pregnant with a singleton or multiples, while a blood test may. Thus, it's likely wise to be patient and get official results from your RE.

What's the Pregnancy Test Like? Any Tips for Managing Nerves?

Most initial pregnancy tests are performed 10 to 14 days after embryo transfer. I still remember the one following my second cycle of IVF: When the 30-second blood test was over, the lyrics of Peggy Lee's classic popped into my head—"Is that all there is?" After months of saving and planning and prepping and treatments, it all came down to a simple stick in the arm and a quick ultrasound to confirm that my uterine lining was sufficiently thick. With that, I was told to expect a phone call from a nurse between 1:00 and 3:00 P.M. At that point, I'd be informed if I was or wasn't in the very early stages of pregnancy. Wow!

While it's not essential for your partner to escort you to your pregnancy test, it's nice for him to keep you company as you await "the call." If the news is bad, you'll want to support each other. If the news is good, you'll want to savor the moment together. What can you expect during that time frame?

Fertility Fact: Celebrity IVFers include Celine Dion, Brooke Shields, Beverly DeAngelo, Cindy Margolis, Wendy Wasserstein, and Courtney Cox.

Nerves, nerves, and more nerves. Is there anything you can do to beat them? For some, listening to classical music or meditating helps, but the majority of IVFers simply resign themselves to a few hours of nail-biting misery. During the wait, I used a fork to reduce my blueberry muffin to crumbs as my husband jabbed at some poor, defenseless scrambled eggs. Then we did some pacing. At 1:33 the phone rang: a chirpy guy selling magazines—arghhh! At 2:07, it rang again: my mom. "No news yet," I informed her rapid-fire, "but I've got to go, the doctor may call soon—bye!" Finally, finally, at 2:57 the phone rang yet again. This time it was Celeste, my favorite nurse from the IVF center. She knew better than to beat around the bush: "I wanted to be the one to give you the news: Your blood test is positive. Congratulations, you've achieved a chemical pregnancy! And the numbers are high, which could mean multiples!"

My husband and I jumped up and down as if we'd won the lottery. After that, we made a conscious effort to rein ourselves in. Although they say there's no such thing as "a little pregnant," in a way there is. It's called a *chemical pregnancy,* which means that the level of human chorionic gonadotropins (HCG) in your blood—that same hormone used to induce ovulation prior to retrieval—is elevated. Make no mistake, achieving a chemical pregnancy is an auspicious sign. It means an embryo (or two) has likely implanted. Still, it's no guarantee that the embryo is healthy or will continue to thrive in the days and weeks to come. For that reason, IVFers are wise to take a position of cautious optimism. My advice: Let yourself get excited—you've earned it!—but bear in mind you've got a ways to go before a successful pregnancy is actually confirmed.

How did my husband and I spend the rest of our day? We shared the news with a few trusted family members. After that, our appetites kicked in so we decided to head over to our favorite restaurant for burgers. On the way, we stopped to admire a tiny, adorable outfit in the window of a baby store. We agreed it was too soon to buy. Still, the mere looking provided a warm rush.

When Am I Really, Truly Considered Pregnant?

During the first few months of pregnancy, HCG levels should double every few days. (A failure to do so often indicates a problem.) It's important to understand, however, that HCG numbers vary widely from woman to woman. The important thing is that they *exponentially rise* as the weeks roll by. An IVFer pregnant with a singleton might get HCG readings along these lines:

- 59 mIU/ml—First Pregnancy Test (10 days post transfer)

- 132 mIU/ml—Second Pregnancy Test (12 days post transfer)

- 2,637 mIU/ml—Third Pregnancy Test (19 days post transfer)

Meanwhile, a woman pregnant with twins would probably have consistently higher numbers. To track these all-important HCG levels, IVFers receive a series of three or more blood tests over the course of several weeks. Although the timetable for pregnancy tests varies from practice to practice, you can expect to receive yours about 10 days to two weeks after your transfer. When does a woman cross the bright line from chemical pregnancy into full-fledged early pregnancy? Answer: when a fetal heartbeat is detected at about six or seven weeks. Was I excited about the results of my initial pregnancy test? Absolutely. But frankly it paled in comparison to the day my RE did an ultrasound and located two bean-sized babies-to-be—both with tiny, steady heartbeats. I still remember his terse words: "OK, it's official: There's a pair . . . you're out of here." "Where to?" I asked with some trepidation. "To a good OB/GYN." Talk about music to my ears. At long last, I was a garden-variety pregnant lady just like all the others!

What If I'm Not Pregnant?

I know from personal experience how hard it is to be told that your pregnancy test has come up negative. Especially cruel is the fact that the news is delivered over the phone, often courtesy of a nurse you may barely know. Crueler still is the reality that you may not be able to sit down with your RE and get answers for several weeks. Following my first failed cycle—I won't lie—I shed a lot of tears. I wish I could tell

---

Fertility Fact: Prior to pregnancy, your uterus is about the size of an apple. But after just six weeks of gestation, it expands to the size of a large grapefruit.

---

you that the experience built character, but I'm not sure about that. I *can* tell you that those horrible feelings—kind of like you've been run over by a freight train—will subside in time. I can also tell you not to give up. Fact: Hundreds of thousands of women with negative pregnancy results go on to achieve healthy pregnancies in future cycles. If you find yourself in this position, turn to Chapter 10. It's stocked with solid strategies, many courtesy of fellow IVFers, for easing the pain and finding the courage to move forward in the face of extreme disappointment.

Can You Tell Me About the Risk of Miscarriage?

Just as miscarriages occur in natural pregnancies, so, too, do they occur in IVF pregnancies. As the graph on the following page indicates, age plays a significant role.

IVF Miscarriage Rates by Age
From the CDC ART Report, 2001

Among women 34 and below, the miscarriage rates are near or below 14 percent. After 34, those rates begin to climb, reaching 30 percent at age 40 and nearly 60 percent by age 44. Why? The culprit is usually older eggs. Sadly, wear and tear can cause chromosomal damage that will inhibit embryos and fetuses from developing beyond a certain point.

Miscarriages are always difficult, but perhaps doubly so for IVFers. Vera, a 39-year-old bank teller, recalls: "One week my HCG test said that I was pregnant, then two weeks later that number plateaued and we knew we had a problem. A few days later, I started to bleed. What a disappointment! After so much time and expense and hope, I had to start over again." Patricia, a 29-year-old accountant, suffered a loss, too: "I was elated when my RE told me I was pregnant with triplets. I knew it was risky, but the idea of an instant family held a lot of appeal. At week six, my RE detected three fetal heartbeats, but by the time I went to my OB/GYN, there were only two. It was sad to lose the one, but I tried to stay strong for my other babies."

Patricia's experience is not unique. In the early weeks of pregnancy, it's not uncommon for IVFers to go from carrying three fetuses to two, or from two to one. In most cases, these fetuses are reabsorbed into the uterine tissue without any bleeding. Still, losing a baby-to-be, even one no larger than a grain of rice, is a significant event that needs to be grieved. If you find yourself in this position, reach out for help from friends and family, even a therapist. Vera shares, "It took me awhile to get over the miscarriage I had during my first cycle. But talking to a counselor really helped me process my emotions and gave me the strength to try again. I'm happy I did because now I have Zach."

A Final Word on the Waiting Room

I opened this chapter with a word about the waiting room. It seems only fitting to close with one, too. As mentioned, the diverse group of women in my IVF waiting room helped me get through my morning tests and even look forward to them. Their warm smiles, words of wisdom, tales from the trenches, and senses of humor made me feel like I belonged. And gave me strength. Although it's certainly not mandatory, I encourage you to meet, greet, and befriend other IVFers. They can help you. Chances are, you can help them, too.

Despite this advice, I caution you to resist comparing notes in too much detail. Why? One of you might get hurt. Consider Robyn's story, a 37-year-old dietician: "I became instant friends with a woman named Gina who always showed up at 7:05 A.M. on the dot, just as I did. At first, it was great—we had so much in common. We were the same age and had the exact same FSH and protocol. But the playing field didn't remain level for the duration. At egg retrieval, she had 30 eggs to my 10. On top of that, she had 20 embryos rated excellent while I had only 2. She was nice as pie about everything. Still, comparing notes, and coming up short, made me feel like a loser. One day, I went straight home and fell on my bed and sobbed—convinced my cycle would be a bust."

The epilogue: Both Robyn *and* Gina achieved pregnancies. Today their children are nearly three and—more coincidences!—in love with watermelon, the color red, and Elmo. Things worked out well in the end. Still, Robyn regrets her decision to share too much and unwittingly turn a great friendship into a quasi–horse race. "If I could give one piece of advice," she says, "It's to keep the specifics of your cycle private. That way, neither of you will feel inadequate. Don't forget it only takes one healthy egg to have a baby."

Chapter 10

To Try Again?

℺

When a Cycle Fails

For most, a failed cycle of IVF is pretty damn heartbreaking. After expending so much time, money, energy, and hope, the chance for a baby has seemingly ended with one simple blood test, one short phone call. Nadine, a 37-year-old reading specialist, remembers her disappointment: "I thought I was mentally prepared for the possibility of not being pregnant, but I guess I wasn't. When the nurse phoned and said I should stop taking progesterone and expect my period within a few days, I kind of lost it. I'm a pretty private person, but I burst into tears—loud, ugly, embarrassing tears. The nurse tried to comfort me as best she could, but what could she say? I felt awful."

I can relate. Having experienced a failed cycle myself, I can personally report that the news of a negative pregnancy test is extremely depressing. As IVF wears on, hope rises like the mercury in a thermometer and we can almost feel that baby in our arms. To have those hopes dashed in an instant is difficult to accept. *It's just not fair!* is the well-intentioned refrain of many a friend and family member. But being reminded of that fact brings little comfort. After all, you're not interested in pondering life's injustice, you just want a baby.

This chapter is here to help you achieve that important goal despite your deep disappointment. In it, you'll find tools for handling the onslaught of emotions you'd likely experience following an unsuccessful cycle. It explains what to expect during the requisite follow-up appointment with your RE as well as the process of undergoing a "frozen" cycle. Additionally, it offers words of wisdom from a variety of IVFers who faced failure and persevered to become joyous parents. So keep reading. It's my sincere hope that these pages will enable you to better manage this difficult time and take the necessary steps to hold that baby in your arms—soon.

Tips for Coping with the No-Baby-Yet Blues

If you've turned to this section following a negative pregnancy result, let me tell you how sorry I am. I remember how much it hurts. If you're anything like me, you're probably lying on the couch, horizontal with disappointment. In addition, some less obvious emotions may be rearing their ugly heads, including frustration (because the procedure didn't work), anger (because the best efforts of your IVF clinic failed), jealousy (because fellow IVFers did achieve pregnancies), exhaustion (because the process took a hell of a lot out of you), and panic (because you're not sure you have the wherewithal to try again). While such reactions aren't particularly cheery, they are pretty valid. And for many, they're a necessary rite of passage. The first step to regaining hope—which you so deserve!—is coming to terms with your head-to-toe sorrow. So let the tears flow. In my opinion, facing those feelings, and resisting the temptation to sweep them under the carpet, is an important part of the healing process.

Another part of the healing process is sharing the news with a few trusted loved ones. My advice is to reserve your most uncensored reactions for your partner. Chances are he's feeling pretty bad, too. Spend some quality time together—crying, yelling, cursing. But don't forget the hugging, holding, soothing. You could both probably use some unconditional support just about now. Isabelle, a 32-year-old Web page designer, recounts: "My husband's a caretaker. When we first got the news that our cycle didn't work, the focus was on me and he was there 100 percent. But the next day when he announced he was heading to bed early without watching his beloved

Yankees in game one of the World Series, I knew he was hurting a lot, too. So I joined him in bed, asking if it was OK to put the game on the radio. He said yes. Then we listened, held hands, and cried a little. Going through those emotions together wasn't a cure-all, but it really helped."

Friends and family members can help, too. Struggling with infertility has an insidious way of making women feel stigmatized, set apart, lonely. No, you needn't tell the world about your fresh disappointment, but discussing your experience with a few key people will probably make you feel a lot less isolated. When my cycle failed, I shared my news with my mother and siblings plus a couple close girlfriends. Most offered just the right words to buoy my spirit. Nevertheless, it's wise to steel yourself for the occasional insensitive remark. For example, a confidante of mine commented, "Everything happens for a reason." While that might be true, it wasn't what I wanted to hear at the moment. Still, I swallowed my resentment, filed the statement away, and took it for what it was—a heartfelt attempt to ease my pain. When you're feeling low, the last thing you need is to be pissed off at an important person in your life. For that reason, it often makes sense to try to focus on a comment's intent, rather than its content. When it comes to friends and family, what really matters is that they care.

What other advice can I offer? Take extra good care of yourself and your partner during this challenging time. As mentioned earlier in this book, it is sometimes human nature—especially among couples with infertility problems—to add insult to injury by withholding creature comforts in response to bad news. We cancel plans with pals, forgo movies and concerts, stop exercising, and essentially get by on bread and water. While it's natural to want to take things slow after a failed cycle, cutting yourself off from the stuff that you love will probably only serve to make you more depressed. Thus, it's wise to engage in some of your favorite activities—whether that's sketching or shopping or cooking or strolling in the park. Sure, it may feel a little forced at first, but returning to your normal routine will help remind you of the riches life has to offer. And for those who can't seem to shake the sadness, consider getting help in the form of therapy or a support group. (Your IVF practice or local chapter of Resolve should be able to furnish quality referrals.)

Give yourself permission to feel lousy, but also to heal. In the hours following my negative pregnancy result, I felt really, really crappy—as if I'd been flattened by a freight train. In those moments, I believed that I would never feel normal again, let alone find myself in a fit state of mind to pursue IVF. But with each day that passed, I took one baby step toward feeling better. And, after a couple weeks, while I wasn't jumping for joy, I was myself again. What's more, I was ready to consider the possibility of a new cycle.

My experience isn't unique. Many of the IVFers I've interviewed for this book report a similar trajectory of healing. First you fall apart, then you pick yourself up and make a new plan. Shannon, a 30-year-old lab technician, recalls: "At first, when the in vitro failed, I thought no way will I go through this again and I was very vocal about it. The pain was so fresh. But after a month, I felt stronger so I said to my husband, 'What do you think of trying again?' Having taken my initial statements at face value, he was a little shocked at my turn-around. But he was totally thrilled to hear it. Now, I'm pregnant." As Shannon's story illustrates, try to avoid talk of abandoning your goal of a baby until you've recovered from the disappointment. The truth is you may feel very differently in a few short weeks—especially if your RE thinks it makes good sense to try again. Often, there is much cause for optimism. Fact: Hundreds of thousands of couples who fail at their first IVF, including myself, achieve success in subsequent cycles.

What to Expect During Your Follow-up Appointment

One of the most difficult aspects of a failed round of IVF is that the bad news is usually delivered over the phone by a nurse—one who may have been only peripherally involved in your treatment. Chances are this nurse will be furnished with your test results, but seldom any information about what went wrong. I still remember the phone call I received informing me of my negative pregnancy results. Even through the blur of bitter disappointment, I wanted to know why. If your cycle was unsuccessful, chances are you'll feel the burning need to connect with your RE right away for answers. That's a reasonable response. If a nurse delivers your results, ask her to help arrange a call from your RE. In my opinion, that's a reasonable request. But don't expect too much from that initial conversation. As bad as your doctor may feel about your outcome, the discussion will likely be short and not terribly illuminating. Why? Most physicians will simply need more time to study what went wrong and develop a new protocol that might have more success.

As a result, REs tend to save most of their commentary for the follow-up appointment, which is usually scheduled about two to six weeks after a cycle's completion. By then, they've had an opportunity to carefully peruse the data in your file and "process" their opinions. Follow-up appointments aren't fun, but they're often informative, even encouraging. Your forecast for future attempts may be a lot rosier than you think! Therefore, I don't recommend putting it off for too long. However, I do recommend waiting until you're feeling sturdy enough to have an open dialogue. Rosie, a 36-year-old patent attorney, told me: "When I didn't get pregnant during my first cycle, I was pretty crushed. But I needed time to regroup and heal emotionally before sitting down and hearing the details about what may have gone wrong. So, I waited four weeks to have my follow-up appointment. That worked out well. By that time, I was ready, willing, and able to hear whatever my doctor had to tell me."

Should your partner escort you on this visit? Absolutely. Like many elements of IVF, the follow-up appointment can be emotionally draining and it's likely you'll need each other's support. Plus, having both of you present will help you capture must-know information. How? One of you can act as the dutiful scribe, as the other takes the lead on asking questions. And while we're on the topic of questions, what exactly should you ask? My advice is to take a few minutes the night before to jot down your queries, which may include:

Questions for the
Follow-up Appointment

1. *What can you tell us about the quality of our eggs, sperm, and embryos? Could one or all of these have been an issue for us?*

2. *In your assessment, what's the most likely explanation for why our cycle failed?*

3. *Do you think it makes sense for us to try again?*

4. *In your opinion, what are our ballpark chances of succeeding in a future cycle?*

5. *If we try again, would you change our protocol? How?*

6. *Are there any additional tests we should have to troubleshoot for undiagnosed factors?*

7. *Are there any special therapies we should consider?*

8. *Is it important that we pursue treatment right away or can it wait several months or even a year?*

9. *Optional: May we have a photocopy of our records?*

10. *Optional (for those with frozen embryos): Does a frozen cycle hold promise for us?*

Follow-up appointments typically run about a half hour to 45 minutes. Will your RE have all the answers? Probably not. The truth is some cases are easier to evaluate than others. Issues related to poor-quality eggs and/or embryos are frequently quite apparent. Medication regimens are sometimes clearly too aggressive or not aggressive enough. Oftentimes, however, the cause of a failed cycle is less evident.

Nevertheless, the best REs work hard to narrow the field to possible factors. They may, for example, suggest further testing to zero in on an undetected antibody disorder that's blocking implantation. They may float the idea of performing Preimplantation Genetic Diagnosis in a future cycle to check each embryo for chromosomal damage. And if you're doing IVF because of tubal problems, they may even ask you to consider the possibility of surgery on your tubes. Why? When a fallopian tube is blocked at the end it often accumulates fluid; this is called a *hydrosalpinx*. Because the same fluid can enter the uterus and create a toxic environment for developing embryos, women with this condition can have trouble sustaining IVF pregnancies. As a result, some practices advocate laparoscopic surgery to sever the tubes. New research shows that success rates for women who had the procedure are about 50 percent higher than their counterparts!

Bottom line: Good physicians do more than shrug their shoulders. No, you can't expect them to be omniscient like those all-knowing narrators in your favorite novels. When it comes to failed cycles, some mystery will always remain. But you *should* expect your RE to be actively engaged in your case. You *should* expect your RE to level with you regarding your chances of success in a future attempt. And, if it makes sense to try again, you *should* expect your RE to make a concerted effort to improve your odds of conceiving—even if that amounts to little more than fine-tuning your existing protocol or simply stating, "I think we should stick with your current treatment plan and here's why." The fact is, not all IVF practices are created equal. Some have far superior success rates than others, and that's attributable, in large part, to the effective micro-management of each patient's unique circumstances.

If you're dissatisfied with your current doctor's handling of your case you may want to consider seeking a second opinion. In a way, this could be a win-win move. Either that new practice will confirm that your current center is doing a good job (which will bring peace of mind) or they'll suggest an alternative protocol. Then, the choice is yours. Nancy, a 36-year-old newspaper reporter, shared her predicament: "I underwent two failed cycles with one center. They were pleasant enough, but my RE was kind of dismissive and didn't seem too interested in trying to figure out how to make things work. So, I decided to check out another clinic across town. It took a little energy, but was totally worth it. The RE there took one look at my records and had a completely different game plan. What he said made sense so I decided to make the leap. It was a gamble, but now I'm three months pregnant!"

Making a Plan
to Move Forward

The decision to try IVF again need not be made overnight. In fact, most REs advise that you wait at least a month or two before pursuing a new cycle, anyway. Why? This essential time frame provides both mind and body a much-needed respite. That being said, women over 37 or those with diminished ovarian reserves shouldn't put off treatment for too long. As mentioned previously, each month that passes subtly reduces fertility. Therefore, although it makes good sense to postpone trying again for several months, several years is probably not a great idea.

Fertility Fact: Because cryopreservation is a relatively new technology, REs don't know how long embryos can actually survive in a frozen state. They do know, however, that a handful of patients have achieved healthy pregnancies after thawing embryos that were frozen for more than 10 years.

But how do you proceed if you're not certain you even ought to proceed? To make a sound decision, it's wise to have one of those good old, partner-to-partner sit-downs that I'm forever mentioning. Choose a quiet time when both of you are feeling calm, open-minded, and receptive to listening. I don't mean to suggest that such discussions are the equivalent of Mid East peace talks. Still, they can get pretty heated. After all, you and your partner may have diametrically opposed views about what your next step should be. One of you, for example, may favor tapping the frozen embryos you have on hand, while the other prefers to pursue a fresh cycle. One of you may be ready to consider using a donor egg, while the other can't abide the idea. One of you may adore your current RE, while the other is ready to seek a second opinion. And one of you may want to try IVF again, while the other thinks its time to talk about adoption.

Are there any absolute truths here? No, probably *both* partners' opinions have merit. So how do you arrive at a reasoned decision? In my opinion, a serious look at the facts is a good starting place, so try to have all of them on hand. Then, as tough as it can be, try to open your ears and truly hear out your mate. Chances are he has some sensible things to say. Just as you do. If things get too heated, take a break and resume talks the next day. In most cases, the tried-and-true tools of patience, rationality, listening, and love will help you arrive at the right decision for both of you.

Pursuing a Frozen Cycle

In the previous section, I mentioned that one of the options for moving forward after a failed attempt at in vitro is a so-called *frozen cycle*. Unfortunately, this isn't an option for everybody. Following IVF, many couples don't have enough high-quality embryos left over to justify freezing and storing them. That being said, about a third of them do. For these IVFers, undergoing a frozen cycle can be a godsend. Why? First and foremost, these embryos don't age. That means if a woman's embryo was cryopreserved when she was 30, it will remain 30 even as she blows out the candles on her 40th birthday cake. Plus, the process is far less invasive than a fresh cycle. Because superovulatory drugs are not needed to grow eggs, this taxing step is simply skipped. Here's more good news: The cost of a frozen cycle ranges in price from $1,600 to $4,000, which is far less than a fresh one. Is there a downside to frozen cycles? Yes, they have a 20 percent success rate, about 5 percent lower than those of fresh cycles. Even so, thousands of couples have pursued frozen cycles and brought home warm bundles of joy, who were at no greater risk of birth defects.

How do frozen cycles work? There are two basic variations. The first is called a *natural frozen cycle*. Yes, I know this sounds like an oxymoron, but bear with me. In this scenario, no drugs are required. Instead a simple ovulation kit is used to pinpoint ovulation, then the transfer is planned to occur at roughly the same time an embryo would naturally arrive in the uterus via the fallopian tubes. The great thing about this process is that it's truly minimally invasive. The second variation, sometimes referred to as a *uterine-primed frozen cycle,* is far more common, and it does require a few medications. In this scenario, a woman is given estrogen and progesterone supplements to "prime" her uterus in an effort to make it extra receptive to incoming embryos. (In some instances Lupron is also prescribed to suppress natural ovulation.)

Fertility Fact: Researchers at the University of Linkoping in Sweden found that couples who had babies via IVF had stronger, more stable families than those who conceived naturally.

In both natural and uterine-primed frozen cycles, the embryos are slowly thawed and nurtured in lab dishes by an embryologist (in much the same way as fresh embryos). About 70 percent of embryos survive the process of going from a frozen to a nonfrozen state. An embryo is considered to "survive" if at least half of its cells are still alive. For example, if an eight-celled embryo still has four cells, that's OK. If all goes well, those four cells will divide to become eight cells, and so on. When is the transfer conducted? That depends on the maturity of the embryos. Since embryos are frozen anywhere from the initial single cell to a 100-cell blastocyst stage, the transfer may happen anywhere from an hour to a few days after the thaw. Brenda, whose embryos were frozen at the blastocyst stage, had her transfer 90 minutes later. Meanwhile, Annie, whose embryos were frozen at the eight-cell stage, had her transfer the next day—a timetable that gave them the opportunity to further mature in the laboratory before entering her uterus. Frozen-cycle transfers are very similar to fresh-cycle ones: The embryos are loaded into a special catheter, then gently injected into the uterus.

Only this time, REs are sometimes willing to transfer slightly higher quantities—if available—to address the slightly lower odds of achieving a pregnancy. As a result, twins and even triplets can and do occur.

In my opinion, frozen cycles are a very good thing because they offer couples a second and sometimes even a third chance to achieve a pregnancy from a single round of in vitro. Brandy, a 30-year-old homemaker, agrees: "I was pretty upset when my fresh cycle failed, but the silver lining was that I was able to freeze six high-quality embryos. The frozen cycle wasn't a cakewalk, but it was a lot less stressful than the first one. And I got pregnant! My daughter is now two and it still freaks me out to think that she spent six months as a teeny tiny frozen embryo. She's truly my little miracle!"

A Final Word on Trying Again

In this book, I've spent a lot of time talking about how to make IVF work. In cases in which egg or sperm quality is poor, there's the option of getting a donor. And in cases where a woman's uterus can't sustain a pregnancy, there's the possibility of relying on a gestational surrogate. But these choices are not right for everyone. The truth is some couples are wise to discontinue treatment, for either personal reasons or poor prognoses. Connie, a 42-year-old family therapist, remembers her experience: "I did two rounds of IVF. One failed and the other resulted in a miscarriage. Both experiences took a lot out of me. It was hard to hear my RE say that my next step should be an egg donor. Not that I have an issue with egg donors—one of my best friends relied on one, and her baby's wonderful, a real blessing. But when my husband, Luke, and I discussed the possibility, we found ourselves hesitating. We were tired of technology, tired of unknowns. And after a great deal of soul-searching we decided that, as much as we wanted a child, we didn't need one to be complete. After all, we have much to be thankful for. We both have large, loving extended families and plenty of nieces and nephews to spoil. Plus, we have stimulating careers, tons of interests, a gorgeous apartment in New

York City, and, most importantly, each other. Did we arrive at our decision to lead a child-free life overnight? No, it took many, many months. But we feel good about it. It's the right choice for us."

Sonia, a 44-year-old painter, and her husband, Kenny, arrived at a different decision: "After our third cycle of IVF failed, I was 42 and it made sense to call it quits. Coming to terms with the reality that we wouldn't have a biological baby took time and I was pretty disillusioned. But after a while, I regained my resolve to be a parent and one day I said to my husband, 'I think we should adopt.' He was a little surprised, but totally over the moon—he'd been a proponent of adoption all along. As odd as it sounds, I'm glad we pursued in vitro. I didn't want to look back on my life and say, 'What if we'd tried IVF?' Giving it our best shot gave me closure and prepared me to move on. Like in vitro, the adoption process took a lot of energy and focus. But we were determined. And now we have a nine-month-old daughter from Guatemala. Our state of mind? Sheer joy! She's amazing and brilliant and beautiful and totally, totally our kid. I know it sounds sort of new agey, but I do believe that of all the babies on the planet this is the one that was meant to be ours."

Sonia is not alone in her thinking. Remarkably, many of the couples I interviewed for this book report a similar sense of destiny regarding their children—whether those children came courtesy of traditional IVF, IVF with the helping hand of a sperm or egg donor, or by way of an adoption agency. "This is the little boy that was made for my arms . . . look how perfectly he fits!" squealed my friend Gretchen, a glowing new mom at the age of 42. I won't bother to share the details of her fertility tale. At the moment, it's not that important. Suffice it to say she is right: Her ebony-haired infant is fast asleep and a perfect fit indeed.

At the close of this book, I want to tell you not to give up on your dream of a child, if a child is what you truly desire. Yes, the pursuit of parenthood can be a challenge, and for some a lengthy and difficult journey. But determination usually breeds success. And when you nuzzle that new baby—regardless of how long the process took or the manner in which your goal was achieved—all will be very, very right with the world.

Glossary

Acupuncture: The Chinese practice of inserting tiny needles into specific regions of the body to relieve pain, cure disease, or increase fertility.

Ampule: A small sealed bottle that holds a solution for hypodermic injection.

Antibodies: Substances produced by a person's immune system that ward off infection by attacking foreign materials entering the body.

Anti-Sperm Antibodies: Substances produced by a male or female's immune system that reduce fertility by attacking sperm, causing it to clump together and/or die.

Antral Follicles: Immature but developing follicles that likely contain eggs.

Assisted Hatching: A process in which the shell-like covering of an early embryo, called the *zona pellucida,* is chemically or mechanically thinned before embryo transfer to help facilitate the hatching process and improve the likelihood of implantation.

Assisted Reproductive Technology (ART): A family of medical procedures that rely on advanced technology to achieve fertilization and pregnancy without intercourse. These include in vitro fertilization (IVF), gamete intrafallopian transfer (GIFT), and zygote intrafallopian transfer (ZIFT).

Basal Body Temperature (BBT) Chart: A day-by-day body temperature chart that helps pinpoint if and when ovulation is occurring.

Blastocyst: An "advanced" embryo containing 64 or more cells that is ready to implant in the uterine lining. This embryonic state usually occurs about five days after fertilization.

Catheter: A thin, flexible tube that gets inserted into the body for the purpose of injecting or withdrawing fluid.

Centers for Disease Control and Prevention (CDC): This federal agency publishes the *Assisted Reproductive Technology Success Rates,* a report enabling consumers to compare the annual success rates of nearly 400 IVF clinics across the country.

Cervical Culture: The process of obtaining and culturing secretions from the cervix to check for the presence of fertility-reducing sexually transmitted diseases, including chlamydia and gonorrhea.

Cervical Mucus: This mucus, produced by the cervix, plays a key role in transporting sperm to the fallopian tubes.

Cervix: The lowermost part of the uterus that opens into the vagina.

Chemical Pregnancy: A "positive" pregnancy test result triggered by an elevated level of human chorionic gonadotropin (HCG) in the blood, but not yet substantiated by ultrasound and/or the detection of a fetal heartbeat.

Chlamydia: A sexually transmitted bacterial infection that, if left untreated, can lead to damaged fallopian tubes and/or pelvic inflammatory disease (PID).

Chromosomes: Minuscule structures in the nucleus of every cell that carry an individual's genetic coding. Chromosomal abnormalities often result in miscarriages or congenital defects.

Clomiphene Citrate: A widely used type of fertility medication, taken orally and used to stimulate ovulation. Brands include Clomid and Serophene.

Consolidated Omnibus Budget Reconciliation Act (COBRA): A 1986 law that guarantees employees who lose their jobs the right to extend their medical coverage for up to 18 months, provided they pick up the monthly payments.

Cryopreservation: The process of freezing embryos or sperm for possible future use.

Dehydroepiandrosterone Sulfate (DHEAS): Excessive levels of this male hormone in women can cause fertility problems. It is often associated with polycystic ovarian syndrome.

Diethylstilbestrol (DES): Commonly prescribed in the 1950s and 1960s to prevent miscarriage, this synthetic estrogen was later found to cause infertility in the offspring of the women who took it. The use of DES during pregnancy was banned in 1971.

Ectopic Pregnancy: A pregnancy that occurs when an embryo implants outside the uterus, usually in the fallopian tubes.

Egg: The female reproductive cell. Also called an *ovum.*

Egg Donation: When a third-party female agrees to undergo stimulation with superovulatory medication, then donate the harvested eggs to another woman—the "intended mother"—to help her achieve a pregnancy via IVF.

Egg Retrieval: The second step of the IVF process, which entails inserting a long needle through the vagina to harvest ripe eggs from the ovaries.

Embryo: Term used to describe a fertilized egg up until about the eighth week of pregnancy.

Embryo Adoption: Programs overseen by adoption agencies that enable couples to receive frozen embryos donated by former IVFers from across the country. This source of embryos follows a traditional adoption model.

Embryo Donation: Programs overseen by IVF clinics that enable couples to receive frozen embryos donated by former patients.

Embryo Transfer: The fourth step of the IVF process, which involves using a special syringe to inject the embryos directly into the uterus.

Embryologist: An M.D. or Ph.D. who specializes in the development of embryos.

Endometrial Biopsy: A test that takes place around day 21 of a woman's cycle in which a small sample of tissue is removed from the uterine wall. The tissue is then evaluated for thickness and receptivity to incoming embryos.

Endometrium: The interior lining of the uterus—otherwise known as the *uterine wall*—in which embryos implant.

Endometriosis: A condition in which bits of the endometrium grow outside the uterus causing painful periods, excessive bleeding, scarring, and sometimes damage to the fallopian tubes and/or ovaries.

Epididymis: The long, tightly coiled, tubular reservoir in which sperm matures prior to ejaculation.

Estradiol: A type of estrogen produced by developing ovarian follicles. During the egg-growing phase of IVF, estradiol levels are measured to get a fix on the quantity and maturity of a patient's egg-containing follicles.

Estrogen: An essential group of female hormones primarily produced by the ovaries.

Fallopian Tubes: Two four-inch-long tubes—connecting the ovaries and uterus—in which natural fertilization takes place.

Family and Medical Leave Act (FMLA): A law, passed by Congress in 1993, that guarantees up to 12 weeks of unpaid leave to employees coping with serious medical issues, such as IVF or the birth of a baby.

Fertilization: When a sperm penetrates an egg, fusing their genetic material.

Fetus: The term used to describe a developing baby from the eighth week of pregnancy until birth.

Fibroid: A benign growth that develops in or on the uterine wall. Although not cancerous, it can cause bleeding, pain, and reduced fertility.

Fimbria: The fingerlike projections at the entrance to the fallopian tubes that catch the released egg during ovulation, then gently sweep it inside for possible fertilization.

Flexible Spending Account: A special account, available at many large companies, in which a portion of an employee's pretax income is set aside to be used for medical expenses.

Follicles: Tiny, blisterlike sacs in the ovaries that house ripening eggs.

Follicle-Stimulating Hormone (FSH): A hormone that stimulates follicle growth and egg development. It is also a key ingredient in all superovulatory drugs.

Fragmentation: Minuscule bits of the cytoplasm that form beadlike blobs on developing embryos. Although about 80 percent of embryos contain some degree of fragmentation, high levels appear to impede implantation.

Fresh Cycle: When fresh, "never-frozen" embryos are used in a cycle of IVF.

Frozen Cycle: When frozen embryos are thawed, then used in a cycle of IVF.

Genetically Engineered Superovulatory Drugs: A new breed of lab-generated medications, derived in part from hamster ovaries, which are often used to stimulate follicle growth during IVF. Available brands include Follistim and Gonal F.

Gestational Surrogate: A woman who agrees to carry a child for another woman, but is neither the genetic nor intended parent.

Gamete Intrafallopian Transfer (GIFT): A procedure in which eggs are retrieved from a woman, mixed with sperm, then promptly transferred into her fallopian tubes via laparoscopy.

Gonadotropins: Hormones—namely, follicle-stimulating hormone (FSH) and luteinizing hormone (LH)— that stimulate a man's testicles to produce sperm and a woman's ovaries to produce eggs.

Gonadotropin-Releasing Hormone: A "messenger hormone" that stimulates the production of follicle-stimulating hormone (FSH) and luteinizing hormone (LH).

Gonadotropin-Releasing Hormone Agonist: A group of fertility medications that suppress ovulation in order to set the stage for egg growth using superovulatory drugs. The most commonly used brand in the United States is Lupron.

Gonadotropin-Releasing Hormone Antagonist: A new class of fertility medications that rapidly suppress ovulation and are sometimes used in place of Lupron during IVF. The two brands now available in the United States are Antagon and Centrotide.

Gonorrhea: A sexually transmitted infection caused by bacteria.

Hamster–Sperm Penetration Test: A test in which human sperm are combined with hamster eggs to assess their ability to penetrate human eggs.

Hormones: Chemicals produced by the endocrine gland, which travel through the body and play a major role in reproduction.

Human Chorionic Gonadotropin (HCG): This hormone, derived from the urine of pregnant women, is given in injection form to female IVFers to trigger the final maturation of their follicles in preparation for egg retrieval. Additionally, HCG is measured during early pregnancy tests; elevated levels suggest that an embryo—or more—has implanted. Available brands include Pregnyl and Profasi.

Human Menopausal Gonadotropin: This group of superovulatory drugs, derived from the urine of post-menopausal women, is often used during IVF to stimulate egg growth. Available brands include Bravelle and Repronex.

Hydrosalpinx: A fluid-filled bulge in the fallopian tubes that can reduce fertility.

Hysterosalpingogram (HSG): A diagnostic test involving X-rays and the injection of a special dye into the uterus to check for abnormalities and blockages of the fallopian tubes.

Hysteroscopy: A diagnostic test in which a small, telescopelike instrument is inserted through the cervix to check the inside of the uterus for fertility-reducing abnormalities such as fibroids and polyps.

Implantation: When an embryo embeds itself in the uterine lining.

Infertility: The inability of a person or couple to achieve and/or sustain a healthy pregnancy.

Intracytoplasmic Sperm Injection (ICSI): A common IVF procedure in which a single sperm is injected directly into an egg to shortcut the fertilization process.

Intramuscular Injections: Shots that get injected into muscle and make use of a one-and-a-half-inch needle.

Intrauterine Insemination (IUI): A procedure in which specially pre-pared sperm is injected into the uterus at ovulation time in order to achieve a pregnancy.

In Vitro Fertilization (IVF): A multi-step process in which a woman's eggs are grown with the aid of superovulatory drugs, retrieved from her ovaries at their peak, fertilized with sperm in lab dishes, then transferred to her uterus in order to achieve a pregnancy.

Karyotyping: Evaluation of the chromosomes to locate abnormalities that may be contributing to pregnancy loss.

Laparoscopy: A surgical procedure in which a small, telescopelike instrument is inserted just under the navel to examine the ovaries, fallopian tubes, and exterior of the uterus for signs of fertility-reducing abnormalities such as endometriosis or scar tissue. If problems are found, they can sometimes be surgically corrected on the spot.

Luteinizing Hormone (LH): This key hormone, released by the pituitary gland, stimulates the ovaries to mature eggs.

Male Factor: When the male partner is responsible for a couple's infertility problems.

Menopause: The phase of a woman's life in which her ovarian reserve is depleted and she ceases to menstruate.

Menstrual Cycle: The time span between menstrual periods. Average cycles last 28 to 31 days with ovulation occurring about midway through.

Micro Epididymal Sperm Aspiration (MESA): The extraction of sperm from the epididymis for use in IVF.

Microsurgery: Delicate surgery performed under magnification using very small instruments.

Miscarriage: Premature ending of a pregnancy.

Mock Embryo Transfer: A trial procedure in which a catheter is inserted through the cervix to simulate an embryo transfer. This quick step helps REs plan for the actual transfer.

Morphology: In the case of sperm, this term refers to their size and structure.

Motility: In the case of sperm, this term refers to their ability to effectively swim forward.

Obstetrician-Gynecologist (OB/GYN): A doctor who specializes in issues related to female reproduction and pregnancy.

Ovarian Hyperstimulation Syndrome (OHSS): Excessive stimulation of the ovaries due to superovulatory drugs. Extreme cases can lead to blood clots, twisted ovaries, and kidney damage or failure.

Ovarian Reserve: The quantity and quality of eggs that remain in the ovaries.

Ovaries: Two almond-shaped organs responsible for storing and releasing eggs.

Ovulation: When an egg (or eggs) is released from the ovaries. Ovulation generally occurs about halfway through a woman's menstrual cycle.

Pap Smear: A test involving the removal of cells from the cervix to screen for cancer.

Pelvic Inflammatory Disease (PID): This infection of a woman's pelvic organs—usually caused by sexually transmitted disease—often leads to reduced fertility.

Placenta: The organ that connects mother and fetus, providing both nourishment and oxygen to the developing baby.

Polycystic Ovarian Syndrome (PCOS): This fertility-reducing condition, caused by a hormonal imbalance, is characterized by infrequent periods and the development of multiple ovarian cysts. It can often be successfully addressed with IVF.

Polyp: A growth on an internal organ, usually benign.

Postcoital Test (PCT): A test used to assess the compatibility of a woman's cervical mucus and her partner's sperm.

Preimplantation Genetic Diagnosis (PGD): The testing of embryos (and sometimes eggs) to check for chromosomal abnormalities prior to implantation.

Premature Ovarian Failure (POF): The ceasing of menstruation due to egg depletion before the age of 40.

Premenstrual Syndrome (PMS): A group of unpleasant symptoms—including mood swings, headaches, water retention, and breast tenderness—that are associated with the onset of menstruation.

Progesterone: A hormone that helps enrich the uterine lining, maximizing the chances of successful implantation. For that reason, progesterone supplements are an important component of the IVF protocol.

Prolactin: An excess of this milk-producing hormone can reduce fertility by disrupting ovulation.

Prolonged Coasting: A protocol occasionally employed during IVF to avoid severe ovarian hyperstimulation syndrome. In this protocol, Lupron is continued, superovulatory drugs are ceased, and the HCG shot and egg collection phase of IVF are delayed until estradiol readings are lowered to safe levels.

Protocol: The specific treatment plan developed for an individual patient.

Reproductive Endocrinologist (RE): An obstetrician-gynecologist who specializes in reproductive medicine.

Resolve: A national nonprofit organization dedicated to helping people cope with and overcome infertility via a national helpline, infertility magazine, RE and therapist referrals, and scores of support groups.

Selective Reduction: A medical procedure used to terminate an early-stage fetus (with an injection of potassium chloride) in order to help safeguard the health of the other fetus or fetuses.

Semen: The combination of sperm, seminal fluid, and reproductive secretions that get released during male ejaculation.

Semen Analysis: A test to assess sperm quantity and quality.

Sexually Transmitted Disease (STD): A disease, such as gonorrhea or chlamydia, that is spread by sexual contact.

Shared-Risk Plans: A new breed of payment plan that enables qualifying couples to purchase a "package" of three or four IVF cycles at a reduced fee and, if all the cycles fail, to then receive a sizable reimbursement.

Society for Reproductive Technology (SART): The professional society for physicians and laboratory scientists who work in the IVF field.

Sperm: The male reproductive cell that's responsible for fertilizing eggs.

Sperm Bank: A place where numerous samples of cryopreserved sperm are stored and available for purchase.

Sperm Count: The percentage of sperm present in the ejaculate.

Sperm Washing: A technique for removing healthy sperm from the ejaculate in order to secure the best possible specimen for use during intrauterine insemination or IVF.

State-Mandated Insurance: Guidelines for medical insurance that are legally enforced by specific states.

Subcutaneous Injections: Shots that get injected just under the skin, using a half-inch needle.

Superovulatory Drugs: A family of fertility drugs that stimulate the growth of multiple eggs and are a key component of the IVF protocol.

Suppression: The shutting down of natural ovulation, usually with the aid of Lupron, Antagon, or Centrotide, to set the stage for the growth of multiple eggs during IVF.

Testicles: Housed in the scrotum, these male organs are responsible for producing sperm and the hormone testosterone. Also called *testes*.

Testicular Sperm Extraction (TESE): The extraction of sperm from the testicles for use in IVF.

Testosterone: The primary male sex hormone.

Thyroid-Stimulating Hormone (TSH): A hormone that stimulates the release of thyroxine from the thyroid gland. Improper levels point to issues related to the thyroid, which sometimes reduce fertility.

Tubal Ligation: A surgical form of birth control in which a woman's fallopian tubes are severed or obstructed to prevent future pregnancies.

Tubal Ovum Transfer (TOT): This Vatican-approved fertility treatment, which is similar to Gamete Intrafallopian Transfer, is carefully designed to meet the Catholic Church's official stance on sex, masturbation, marriage, and contraception.

Ultrasound: A diagnostic test that uses high-frequency sound waves to create black-and-white pictures of a patient's internal organs—including the uterus, fallopian tubes, and ovaries—which appear on a TV-like screen. Also called a *sonogram*.

Unexplained Infertility: When the source of an individual or couple's infertility cannot be determined through extensive testing.

Urologist: A physician who diagnoses and treats disorders of the male urinary and reproductive organs.

Uterus: A hollow, pear-shaped, muscular organ in which fetuses develop until birth.

Varicoceles: A collection of enlarged veins around the testicles that raise the temperature of the testes and, in so doing, reduce sperm production. Varicoceles are the leading cause of male infertility.

Vas Deferens: The two long tubes in the scrotum that transport sperm from the testes into the ejaculatory ducts of the penis.

Vasectomy: A surgical form of birth control in which the sperm supply is eliminated from the ejaculate.

Vasectomy Reversal: Surgical repair of a previous vasectomy.

Zygote Intrafallopian Transfer (ZIFT): A procedure in which eggs are retrieved from the woman, fertilized with sperm, then promptly transferred into her fallopian tubes via laparoscopy for possible fertilization.

Online Resources

American Infertility Association (www.americaninfertility.org): Information, advocacy, and links related to overcoming infertility.

American Society for Reproductive Medicine (www.asrm.org): A font of IVF data for both REs *and* patients, including a roundup of state-by-state infertility insurance policy.

American Surrogacy Center (www.surrogacy.com): Articles, classified ads, message boards, and more—all dedicated to the important topic of surrogacy.

Centers for Disease Control and Prevention (www.cdc.gov/reproductive health): The *Assisted Reproductive Technology Success Rates,* a 500-plus page document published on the CDC's Web site, enables couples to compare the success rates of nearly 400 clinics nationwide.

Conceiving Concepts (www.conceivingconcepts.com): Tips, fertility products, and a very active chat room.

FertileThoughts (www.fertilethoughts.net): Covers the many fronts of infertility, including in vitro, surrogacy, and adoption.

Fertilitext (www.fertilitext.org): This site, which is sponsored by a chain of drugstores, offers jargon-free IVF information with a focus on fertility meds.

FertilityPlus (www.fertilityplus.org): A friendly site full of advice written by patients, for patients.

Ferti.Net (www.ferti.net): Infertility news from around the world.

InterNational Council on Infertility Information Dissemination (www.inciid.org): Loads of up-to-date data related to infertility plus bulletin boards and online chats featuring prominent REs.

Internet Health Resources (www.ihr.com): This portal provides links to dozens of fertility-related sites.

IVF Connections (www.ivfconnections.com): Moving, firsthand accounts from IVFers along with dozens of great bulletin boards.

IVF.net (www.ivf.net): This England-based site posts breaking IVF news from the U.K., the United States, and elsewhere.

National Adoption Information Clearinghouse (www.naic.acf.hhs.gov): The government's clearinghouse for information on adoption-related issues.

National Certification Commission for Acupuncture and Oriental Medicine (www.nccaom.org): Features a database to help you locate a licensed acupuncturist in your neck of the woods.

Organization of Parents Through Surrogacy (www.Opts.com): Practical information and support related to all aspects of surrogacy.

Resolve (www.resolve.org): Provides referrals to IVF clinics, infertility therapists, local support groups, and much, much more.

Shared Journey (www.sharedjourney.com): Super chat rooms and solid facts on infertility, miscarriage, surrogacy, child-free living, and adoption.

Snowflakes Embryo Adoption Program (www.Snowflakes.org): Everything you need to know about the process of embryo adoption via the Snowflakes Program.

Society for Assisted Reproductive Technology (www.sart.org): Intended for REs and the patients they serve, this site posts key IVF guidelines and information.

U.S. Department of Labor (www.dol.gov): Offers an explanation of both the Consolidated Omnibus Budget Reconciliation Act (COBRA) and the Family Medical Leave Act (FMLA), two bills relevant to IVFers.

Acknowledgments

A great many people helped me turn an idea—at the outset, just a glimmer in my eye—into the book you are holding. First and foremost, I'm enormously grateful to the dozens of amazing women—and men—who stepped forward to share the intimate details of their IVF experiences. Although their identities have been changed to preserve their anonymity, their stories come through loud and clear. All were candid, courageous, and downright inspiring. Their IVF tales form the heart and soul of this book and, quite simply, I couldn't have done it without them.

I'm also extremely thankful to the many in-vitro doctors who were so generous in setting aside time from their hectic schedules to illuminate the process. A heartfelt thanks to Dr. John Hesla at the Portland Center for Reproductive Medicine, who pored over this manuscript during one of the worst ice storms in Oregon history, offering incisive comments and kind encouragement. I'd like to thank Dr. Brad Kolb, Dr. Jane Frederick, and Rachel Ragoff, R.N., all of Huntington Reproductive Center in Southern California. Thanks, as well, to Dr. Larry Werlin of Coastal Fertility Medical Center in Irvine; Dr. Geoffrey Sher of the Sher Institute for Reproductive Medicine in Las Vegas; Dr. Nicole Noyes of the New York University Program for IVF; Dr. Daniel Stein of the Division of Reproductive Endocrinology and Infertility at St. Luke's Roosevelt in New York City; Dr. David McLaughlin of the Indianapolis Medical Center; and Dr. Jeffrey Boldt of the Southeastern Center for Fertility and Reproductive Surgery in Knoxville.

In addition, my great appreciation goes to Shelley Smith of the Egg Donor Program of Los Angeles; Karen Synesiou, cofounder of the Center for Surrogate Parenting in Encino; and attorney Mary Cedarbade, who clarified the many legal issues relevant to IVF. Therapists with an expertise in infertility are a godsend. Thankfully, I received guidance from two of the best—Los Angeles–based counselor Carole Lieber Wilkins and, in Manhattan, counselor Susan O'Brecht. Special thanks are also in order for IVF consultant Sophia Bellandi and acupuncturist Jill Blakeway.

Now, on to some invaluable folks who helped on the publishing end: Thanks to my excellent editor, Marnie Cochran—first, for taking a chance on a new author; second, for making such savvy recommendations; and third, for being a joy to work with. Sincere thanks to senior project editor Erin Sprague for moving the manuscript forward with alacrity, to copy editor John C. Thomas for his skillful edits, and to designer George Restrepo for creating the perfect book cover. Of course, I'm also indebted to my agent, Richard Curtis of Richard Curtis Associates. All authors should be fortunate enough to be represented by someone as knowing and kind.

Having a close friend who's a doctor *and* an IVFer is like winning the lottery. Lucky me! My old pal Dr. Ingrid Kemperman was able to weigh in on both sides of the in-vitro process. Hugs and kisses to my mom, Sylvia Charlesworth, a sharp-eyed proofreader, whose gifts helped to shape this manuscript, as well as to my cheerleading siblings—Jacqueline, Greg, and Eric. Thank yous wouldn't be complete without mention of my twin sons, Dash and Theo—you kept me ebullient through many weeks of writing. Finally, huge thanks to my husband, Justin Martin, for the tips, edits, support, emergency babysitting sessions, and everything in between.

Index